Defeat Diabetes

33 Effective Strategies To End Diabetes – Before It Ends You

By: Drs. Stephanie and Thomas Chaney

Defeat
Diabetes

33 EFFECTIVE STRATEGIES

To End Diabetes –
Before It Ends You

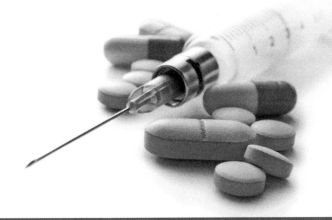

Stephanie J. Chaney, D.C. & Thomas A. Chaney, D.C.

Copyright © 2017: Drs. Stephanie and Thomas A. Chaney, D.C.

All rights reserved. No part of this publication may be reproduced or transmitted in any form or by any means, mechanical or electronic, including photocopying and recording, or by any information storage and retrieval system, without permission in writing from the author, with the exception of a reviewer who may quote brief passages.

All trademarks are the property of their respective companies.

Cover Design by Paul M. Wilson

Cataloging-in-Publication Data is on file with the Library of Congress.

ISBN: Print Book - 978-xxeBook - 978-xx

PROUDLY PRINTED IN THE UNITED STATES OF AMERICA
By Selby Marketing Associates

Disclaimer: This information is intended as a reference volume only, not as a medical manual. The information given here is designed to help you make informed decisions about your health. The author makes no representations or warranties with respect to the accuracy or completeness of the contents of this work and specifically disclaims all warranties, including without limitation warranties of fitness for a particular purpose. No warranty may be created or extended by sales or promotional materials. The advice and strategies contained herein may not be suitable for every situation. This author shall not be liable for damages arising herefrom. This information isn't intended as a substitute for any treatment that may have been prescribed by your doctor. The fact that a doctor, organization, or website is referred to in this work as a citation or source of information doesn't mean that the author endorses the information the organization, the doctor, or website may provide or recommendations it may make. If you suspect that you have a medical problem, we urge you to seek competent medical help.

This book is dedicated to the millions that struggle with Type 2 Diabetes; the persistent and the passionate who have been rendered hopeless, having been provided with only conventional tools and advice to merely 'manage' their disease instead of defeating it.

CONTENTS

INTRODUCTION

As we write this book, it's becoming increasingly clear that the health of this nation, as well as that of the rest of the world, is heading in the wrong direction. An increasing number of patients enter our health care office each year suffering from multiple conditions, complaining of several symptoms, and carrying long lists of medications to address these symptoms. Obesity and diabetes rates continue to increase.

UnitedHealth Group's Center for Health Reform and Modernization predicts that half of the U.S. population will be either pre-diabetic or diabetic by the year 2020.[1] Currently, the Centers for Disease Control and Prevention (CDC) report that 50 percent of the U.S. population has high blood pressure, high cholesterol, or diabetes. Their figures show that as of 2012, 29.1 million Americans suffer from type 2 diabetes while almost one-third of the country (86 million) has pre-diabetes.[2] The cost of handling this load of ill health is an astonishing $174 billion as of 2007, with estimates of more than $200 billion by 2020.[3] The majority of patients seeking medical care for these issues continue to be frustrated with the state of their health and the futile search for long-term solutions.

As doctors, health care practitioners, and patients, we encounter thousands of health products that include supplements, diets, and books each year. Companies market their products as a quick fix for all ills. Upon closer inspection, results often indicate that most health products offer only temporary help, while many offer no help at all. Some products may even be hazardous to your health.

This book isn't about temporary or risky solutions. On the contrary, this book is about safe, healthy, and long-term solutions to modern, chronic, and deadly diseases. If you're searching for a quick fix, you can stop reading now. It doesn't exist.

Throughout our lifetime search for optimal health, we've discovered that there are no shortcuts to establishing and maintaining excellent health. Just like planning for retirement, establishing and maintaining proper long-term health takes goals, a plan, and action. There is no such thing as a "one-size-fits-all health plan"—everyone's health plan should look a little different in order to meet all individual needs. However, there are some core concepts, principles, and ideas that should be a part of every long-term health plan.

Both professional and personal experiences have shown us that when patients implement these core concepts, their health improves dramatically. This book will outline the core concepts, principles, and actions that will not only help you reverse or prevent diabetes, they will help you secure and retain sound health.

When our patients become healthier, their quality of life improves, they become more active, they enjoy more time with their families, and they are happier. When patients regain their health, they become more productive and better able to fulfill their dreams, which ultimately benefits society as a whole. We see patients reverse their type 2 diabetic condition despite the medical monopoly that says it's not likely to happen. Visit www.DiabetesReversalProgram.com to see and hear from some of our patients. You'll also see that if they can do it, you can, too.

The Proof is in the Pudding

You might be wondering, "Why should I pay attention to the information in this book?"

The answer is that results speak for themselves. In our office, we help diabetics reverse type 2 diabetes every day. That means they are able to reduce and eliminate the need for medication while maintaining blood sugar in normal range for the long term. We can share many patient testimonials that show how these results can be achieved with a complete diagnosis of the problems and the right plan to correct them. The tools in this book are grounded in clinical results—results that we've obtained from working with thousands of patients. We aren't researchers or professors, and we aren't connected to pharmaceutical companies. We're clinicians sharing the tools that help real people in our office every day. Here are a few clinical case studies that demonstrate the types of results we see in our clinic.

Case # 1

A 65-year-old female we will call Patty had been diabetic for more than 20 years. She came to us looking for help. Patty, who had been to an endocrinologist and a nutritionist, was diagnosed with neuropathy, sleep apnea, high cholesterol, and high blood pressure in addition to diabetes. A few months before Patty came to see us, the endocrinologist prescribed insulin in addition to the Metformin, Crestor, Toprol, and Losartan Patty was already taking. By the time she got to our office, she was injecting insulin five times a day for a total of 130+ daily units.

This patient felt like her health was spiraling out of control. Her blood sugar continued to increase despite her medications; she felt like a victim unable to stop the downward spiral. Patty said that she was doing everything her doctor and nutritionist recommended—she even hired a personal trainer and was consistently exercising. She was seeing the nutritionist several times a month and following the prescribed diet. Yet, month after month, Patty watched the doctor increase her insulin dose while she continued to take the other medications.

When she came in to see us, we ordered a battery of comprehensive tests that let us find the problems that needed to be addressed—problems the medications weren't solving. Once we got her started on a program, she started seeing results within the first couple of weeks. Her blood sugar and insulin dosage were dropping.

Over the next eight months, we were able to get Patty to the point where she no longer needed insulin, had lost more than 50 pounds, had more energy, was sleeping better, and had a

Hemoglobin A1C (HbA1C) of 6.0 percent. (HbA1C that is greater than 6.4 percent is in diabetic range.) As you can imagine, Patty was very happy with her results. She has since been able to maintain and even improve them since completing her program.

Case # 2

A 27-year-old male we'll call Matt came to our office after having just been hospitalized with blood sugar readings of 500+ (normal blood sugar is 80 to 100). This wasn't the first time Matt had been hospitalized due to high blood sugar. After a couple of days, his hospital team was able to get his blood sugar low enough to release him.

When he came into see us, Matt's sugar reading was still 300+ while on Metformin, Glimepiride, and Januvia for the problem. He was also taking medication for high cholesterol and blood pressure. Matt had changed his diet and was following doctor's orders, but wasn't seeing results. We sent him out for testing that revealed the problems we needed to help him correct. In only three weeks on our treatment plan, Matt's blood sugars were consistently 80 to 100.

Just a few months later, Matt could stop taking all of his medications because he was keeping his blood sugar, blood pressure, and cholesterol all in a normal range. Today, he is no longer considered to be a diabetic.

When you identify the true causes of the problems and correct them, results happen quickly.

Case #3

We had a 64-year-old male, "Don," come to see us out of sheer frustration. He had been diagnosed with type 2 diabetes nine years before. Don was frustrated because he was an active cyclist riding 50-plus miles a week, yet his health continued to decline.

Each time he went to the doctor for a checkup, his situation was worse and the doctor put him on more medications. This didn't make sense to Don because he was so active. His doctor told him to exercise, and that's exactly what he was doing.

By the time we saw him, Don's HbA1C was 8.9 percent and he was taking Metformin, Actos, and Glipizide for his diabetes. He was also taking Digitoxin, Coreg, and Ramipril. We ran a comprehensive set of tests based on blood, urine, saliva, and stool samples. We were able to identify his problems and develop a plan to correct them. In four months of treatment under our care, Don's HbA1C came down to 5.7 percent while only on a low dose of Glipizide, which was eventually eliminated. You can imagine how happy he was!

If You Have Been Told You Can't Reverse Your Type 2 Diabetes, IT'S NOT TRUE!

This book reveals health strategies that many health care professionals don't want you to discover. Unfortunately, within the current health care structure, health problems equal health profits. More sick or ill people mean more visits to a provider, health care jobs, prescribed pharmaceuticals, and lifetime customers dependent on drugs and surgery. All of this means more net profits for the health care industry.

As of this writing, the health care system is currently estimated at almost 18 percent of the gross domestic product of the U.S., with that number predicted to be up to 20 percent by 2020. People requiring medical intervention comprise one of the country's largest industries. Diabetes care, and the diseases and complications associated with it, are a big part of this. Many medical institutions have little incentive to get you healthier or provide a solution that fixes or "cures" the problem, since your illness contributes to their economic growth and survival, especially when it comes to "big pharma." It's more profitable to keep you in the dark, avoid teaching you how to be healthier, and keep you dependent on a system designed to create profit.

Let us also state that we think we have some of the best medical professionals in the world in this country. There is without a doubt a time and place for medical care. However, when it comes to disease prevention and promoting healthy living, the ball gets dropped. The World Health Organization ranks the United States health care system 37th among developed nations, yet we spend more per capita than any other country. We're sure that some of you may be thinking, "My doctor is one of the best and most intelligent and caring doctors out there." Yes, he or she probably is. But traditional doctors are part of a system. They're taught to use conventional tools, medications, and procedures. Unfortunately, these tools aren't designed to promote health or fix the cause of chronic diseases such as diabetes, high blood pressure, and heart disease. What they offer are often just a short-term BAND AID®, if that.

The Conventional Standard of Care

In our office, we see hundreds of patients every month. Most of our diabetic patients come in telling a similar story, one we hear over and over again. This is, or likely will be, your story.

You visited your doctor, maybe only for a routine checkup. Perhaps you were experiencing blurred vision, urinating more frequently, or feeling very thirsty or tired. The doctor ran tests – probably blood work. The blood tests revealed that you had high blood sugar; you were then diagnosed as having type 2 diabetes.

The doctor prescribed your first diabetes pill—Metformin is the most common, with more than 40 million prescriptions written in the U.S. per year. The accompanying lifestyle recommendations—"lose weight, change your diet, and exercise"—are the same across the board. They are vague and usually leave you trying to figure what that really means considering you haven't received specific instructions on how to do it. This is where your journey down the diabetes road begins.

Your doctor instructs you to return for follow-up appointments every few months. This process involves running the same tests periodically to see how you're doing; eventually, a few red flags start waving. Your cholesterol is likely on the rise, requiring a statin prescription. High blood pressure is next—and so is yet another medication for that. We're seeing

WEIGHT ISN'T THE CAUSE OF YOUR DIABETES.

Your weight or fat gain and loss of muscle are due to the functional imbalances that are occurring in your body, including the elevated blood sugars and insulin resistance at the core of your pre-diabetes or diabetes.

This means that you aren't diabetic because you're fat, you're fat because of elevated sugars in the body and what the body has to do to keep blood sugars normal. It's a "chicken or the egg" puzzle, but in this case, the process starts with sugar and insulin levels in the body that are too high. This results in you gaining more fat. This is an important distinction because it dictates how you treat it so you get healthy.

We have treated many "skinny" diabetics, so how can you tell them that weight is causing their disease? Obviously, there are other factors at play.

Moreover, many of the medications prescribed for type 2 diabetes cause weight gain and/or hunger, so medications may be an additional contributing factor to the amount that someone weighs. The good news is that when these functional imbalances are corrected, weight loss becomes easy. Our point is, just losing weight doesn't mean you're correcting the cause of your diabetes and getting healthier. And not every type 2 diabetic is overweight, so it doesn't make sense to say your weight is causing your diabetes.

more and more patients get put on these medications at the very onset of their diabetes diagnosis as a "preventative" measure, even if their cholesterol or blood pressure isn't high yet.

As you go back in for routine checkups, you learn that your original dose of blood sugar medication isn't effective. Your HbA1c is likely more elevated, so the doctor increases the blood sugar medication, and may even add another prescription to the original pill. We see patients coming in on two, three, or even four oral medications for their type 2 diabetes.

Do You Want to Treat the Symptoms or the Cause?

One of the problems with the conventional approach to diabetes is that it doesn't address the cause of the elevated blood sugar—it only treats the symptoms. The patient may in fact need medication to get her blood sugar down initially, but she also needs to address the cause of these health conditions for the long-term or the disease will simply continue to progress.

You eventually max out on the oral medication options so the doctor has no choice but to use the last tool: insulin. Meanwhile, you start to develop complications because insulin worsens the insulin resistance and speeds the progression of this disease. The only thing to do going forward once you're on insulin is to keep increasing the dose. Eventually, you could end up like one of our patients: 35 years old with sugars in the 300s and taking 400 units of insulin each day.

The complications we see related to that include neuropathy in the feet and hands. We saw a patient recently whose feet burned so badly that he was lucky to get two hours of sleep—even while taking three pain medications.

We also see patients with diabetes-related vision problems, including blindness. Some patients have had a heart attack or stroke, since cardiovascular events are very common killers of type 2 diabetics. Kidney failure and limb amputation are part of the equation, too.

We Know What You Have Been Told to Do

Unfortunately, as this process plays out, patients are given little or no real education or tools that help address lifestyle choices that are impacting their health. Most patients come to our office having been told they need to lose weight, start exercising, and change their diet. They are sent to dieticians or nutritionists who give them a cookie-cutter diet that isn't specific to them. Fact is, there's no single "diabetic diet" that's going to work for everyone. What's more, even the general principles that we know work to help get sugars down aren't being taught by these conventional practitioners. In fact, we often find that what patients have been told to eat and drink to help "manage" their diabetes ends up making them worse. Patients come to us frustrated because their lifestyle and diet changes haven't worked, and this is all while they're being given more and more medication for mounting health problems.

Some patients have even been told that they're type 2 diabetic because of their genetics. Their mother and grandmother had it, so they are destined to have it, too. But they aren't tested to see if it truly is a genetic problem or not. It's just an opinion and unfortunately for the patients, they feel at that point there isn't anything they can do about it.

We can tell you from the thousands of patients we have helped that genetics have only been a factor in a very, very small percentage. Still, even with these tough genetic cases, patients can improve. The other consideration is that genes can be influenced and affected by the environment we expose them to, which means that putting all the emphasis on the "gene theory" is a mistake, since genes can be turned on and off by our environment. We don't want you to ever feel like there's nothing that can be done. We feel that this disease and all of the complications that go along with it can be prevented and reversed with the right approach.

One thing is certain to us each time we sit down with a type 2 diabetic: The current conventional standard of care isn't an effective long-term solution for them. The medications aren't fixing the problems, so the disease continues to progress and get worse. If these medications really fixed the problem and the cause of your disease, you wouldn't be expected to stay on them for the rest of your life.

The patients who come to our practice are at various diabetes stages or health levels. Some are much sicker than others. The sicker you are, the more work and time it takes to regain health, so be patient with yourself and seek professional attention if you're suffering from diagnosed conditions such as high blood pressure or high cholesterol in addition to diabetes. You may require advanced individual treatment.

HOW TO USE THIS BOOK

This book is designed to give you action steps that are easy to implement and incorporate into your lifestyle. When you finish reading a section, apply the principle and work out whatever actions are needed to keep that principle a part of your ongoing life, then move on to the next principle and implement as you did the previous one. Go at your own pace, but understand that the more of these principles you're applying at once, the better your results will be—and the more momentum you'll have.

Applying the principles in this book doesn't require special skills, knowledge, or expertise, but some require discipline and willpower. These principles will help guide you to your health goals. If you've implemented most or all of them and you're still having trouble with your blood sugars, look for a health care practitioner who practices "functional medicine" to run more advanced testing to determine what other interventions you may need. They're typically chiropractors, naturopaths, nurse practitioners, or forward-thinking medical doctors.

ARE YOU DIABETIC OR PRE-DIABETIC?

Some confusion persists in the medical world as to whether the condition known as pre-diabetes even exists. We see patients who have been told that they are pre-diabetic or borderline diabetic, but their test results show that they're actually type 2 diabetic. Some are told they're diabetic and put on medications right away without being given the opportunity to make lifestyle changes first.

Let's talk about testing and how these tests help us determine if you're pre-diabetic, type 2 diabetic, or type 1 diabetic.

HbA1c

The majority of patients routinely visit their primary care doctors. During these checkups, the doctor orders tests which typically include blood work. One of the markers in the blood that's checked is the hemoglobin A1C (HbA1C). HbA1C is measured generally every three months because it's a percentage of red blood cells that are damaged by blood sugars and those red blood cells live, on average, three months. You don't have to wait three months to see significant improvement if you take steps to dramatically improve blood sugars. Clinically, we've seen double-digit HbA1c readings come down to the seven-level in as little as four weeks.

The normal functional HbA1C range is between 4.7 percent and 5.7 percent. This is the target range anyone must maintain to stay out of the pre-diabetic or diabetic range. Pre-diabetes is defined by the American Diabetes Association as a patient with HbA1C between 5.8 percent and 6.4 percent. This means that the person has higher than normal blood sugar, but isn't in the diabetic range yet. The diabetic range is HbA1C higher than 6.4 percent. The HbA1C marker is the most commonly used test to determine blood sugar levels. Medication is indicated in the standard of care model when HbA1c reaches 7 percent or higher.

BLOOD GLUCOSE

When you were diagnosed as pre-diabetic or diabetic, you were likely asked by your doctor to start checking your blood sugar. It's important to know your blood sugar level, so if you aren't checking yours, start now. Most diabetics will check their fasting blood sugar first thing in the morning, then check one to four times more throughout the day depending on the severity of their condition. If you don't know how to check your blood sugar or were never given a meter, contact your doctor's office for supplies and instructions. You can also find supplies online at various wholesale diabetes outlets.

The pre-diabetic may also experience symptoms, but these symptoms are more common once the sugars have elevated into diabetic range. Some of these symptoms include increased thirst, frequent urination, lack of energy, frequent illness, blurred vision, slow-to-heal wounds, and numbness or tingling in the hands or feet. Most pre-diabetics have no symptoms, though. Getting tested is the best way to know if your blood sugar is under control and whether you're pre-diabetic or diabetic. Ask your doctor to check your HbA1C the next time you go in for a checkup, or order a home HbA1c test kit or meter to do it yourself.

Other tests can be performed, as well. The fasting plasma glucose test will require you to fast overnight, and then have your blood glucose tested first thing in the morning. Generally, a normal level is 60 to 100 mg/dl, but we find clinically 80 to 100 is ideal. A result between 100 and 125 mg/dl could indicate pre-diabetes. When it's over 125 mg/dl, it could indicate diabetes.

UNDERSTANDING YOUR TEST RESULTS

	Fasting Blood Sugar	HbA1C
Non-Diabetic Range	Less than 100 mg/dl	Less than 5.7%
Pre-Diabetic	100-125 mg/dl	5.7%- 6.4%
Diabetic	126 mg/dl or higher	6.5% or higher

GLUCOSE TOLERANCE TEST

Another test is the oral glucose tolerance test. Just like the plasma glucose test, your fasting blood glucose will be tested. For this test, you'll drink a glucose-rich mixture; two hours later, your blood glucose is measured again. Generally, a normal level is below 140 mg/dl. If it's between 140 and 199 mg/dl, it could indicate pre-diabetes. When it's over 200 mg/dl, it could indicate diabetes.

FASTING INSULIN

Fasting insulin is a great test for anyone suspecting that they may have diabetes, or as a general wellness test. It's rarely done, even if one has diabetes. The body will compensate and do whatever it can to maintain normal blood glucose levels. If sugar goes up to a higher than ideal range, then the pancreas will secrete insulin to help clear sugar out of the blood, forcing it into storage for use later (often as fat in fat cells). One may have normal blood glucose levels for years, but insulin levels may be higher than normal in order to keep these normal blood glucose levels. This often happens long before pre-diabetes or diabetes is diagnosed, so insulin can be one of the earliest markers for blood sugar issues.

Insulin is measured in "microunits per milliliter" (mcU/ml or mIU/ml). There is little agreement on what level is ideal. By some lab standards, measures up to 27 mcU/ml are considered a safe range[5]. Some researchers generally agree that the ideal target range would be 2 to 5 mcU/ml[6]. Fasting insulin levels above 5 mcU/ml can be an indicator of pre-diabetes and insulin resistance, especially in the presence of normal blood glucose values. It can indicate that to maintain sugars in a normal range, you have to secrete higher than ideal amounts of insulin to overcome the insulin resistance.

OTHER

There are several other tests that help distinguish type 1 from type 2 diabetes. These are generally blood markers to assess whether your immune system is attacking the insulin-producing (beta) cells of your pancreas or other enzymes related to pancreas function and insulin production. These include antipancreatic antibodies and glutamic acid decarboxylase enzyme (GAD) antibodies.

A positive result on either test would indicate that you're type 1 or, possibly, a combination of both type 1 and 2. This is referred to as latent autoimmune diabetes in adults (LADA)—more on that later. This is helpful information if you find this out as a pre-diabetic because you can implement early strategies to help slow down the progressive destruction of your pancreas. In some cases, you can avoid being put on insulin.

Generally, you will have been pre-diabetic for some time before developing type 2 diabetes. The good news is that if you have pre-diabetes, you can take several steps to help minimize your risk of getting full-blown diabetes. If you don't take the necessary precautions, your overall health could be at greater risk. Unfortunately, many people think that because they have pre-diabetes instead of diabetes, they don't have to be as cautious about their health. This is simply not the case. This disease process will continue to worsen over time unless you take steps to reverse it.

Recent studies have shown that pre-diabetes can damage the body. This is especially true of the heart and circulatory system. People with elevated sugar levels are also more likely to get cancer, Alzheimer's disease, and other debilitating illnesses. Those with pre-diabetes should be just as aware as their type 2 diabetes counterparts are of certain ailments and illnesses that can occur because of their disease.

Make sure you're doing your part to promote better health. Stay in touch with your doctor to track your HbA1C levels. When you know where they stand, you're more likely to keep your health in check. Without knowing your HbA1C levels, you won't be certain about what you need to work on.

Type 1 Diabetes vs. Type 2 Diabetes

Many of our patients come in confused about the different types of diabetes or have been told they're type 2 diabetic but are actually either type 1 or LADA (type 1.5). Or, they've never been told what type of diabetic they are.

TYPE 1 DIABETES

Type 1 diabetes occurs when the pancreas is producing very little or no insulin because the insulin-producing beta cells have been destroyed. In many cases, it progresses to the point where the diabetic requires insulin injections.

If you're injecting insulin, you aren't necessarily a type 1 diabetic. Many of our type 2 diabetic patients come in on insulin, often as a last resort when oral medications have failed to adequately control rising blood sugars. In fact, roughly 5 percent of those diagnosed with diabetes have type 1.[7]

Type 1 occurs most often in teenagers but can occur in adults and young children, as well. When it occurs in adults, it's referred to as latent autoimmune diabetes in adults (LADA), or type 1.5 diabetes. The 1.5 refers to the likelihood that the adult has both type 1 (non-production of insulin) and type 2 characteristics (insulin resistance). The appropriate testing explained earlier can determine the type you have.

TYPE 2 DIABETES

Type 2 diabetes begins when the body is producing insulin, but experiences problems elsewhere, including insulin resistance. There are many organs, systems, glands, and cells involved in controlling blood sugar. If any are compromised and not functioning the way they should, your body won't be able to regulate your blood sugar. It's estimated that more than 90 percent of the people with diabetes have type 2. It was previously referred to as adult onset diabetes but we are seeing the disease in young adults and children at a high rate, too.

How does your body regulate sugar?

It's important to understand that the pancreas isn't the only gland or organ involved in regulating blood sugar levels because everything involved plays a role in getting your body back on track so you can reverse your diabetes.

Many type 2 diabetics think or have been told that they have a pancreas problem. The vast majority of those we have worked with over the years don't have a pancreas problem at all. There are issues elsewhere in the body that cause a build-up of blood glucose and insulin, which leads to insulin resistance. Here's a general list and description of several major organs and glands involved in regulating blood sugars:

PANCREAS and INSULIN

The pancreas is a gland that is part of both the digestive and endocrine systems. It produces several hormones, including insulin and glucagon.

Insulin is a hormone secreted by pancreas beta cells. It allows the liver and muscles to use glucose for energy and to store it as glycogen for quick use later. Insulin also facilitates glucose storage in fat cells as triglycerides. It also controls other body systems and regulates the amino acid (protein) uptake into cells[8].

Glucagon works in the opposite manner of insulin. It's secreted by the alpha cells of the pancreas and stimulates the release of glucose from storage by causing stored glycogen to be converted back to glucose and released into the blood stream to elevate blood glucose levels.

Insulin and glucagon work together in opposition in a feedback loop to help maintain a steady level of blood sugar. If blood sugar is too high, insulin is secreted. If blood sugar gets too low, glucagon is secreted.

The high levels of insulin that result from elevated blood sugars and insulin resistance found in both pre-diabetics and diabetics have been associated with several disease processes in addition to type 2 diabetes: obesity, cancer, chronic inflammation, hypertension, atherosclerosis, and strokes.[9, 10, 11, 12, 13]

INSULIN RECEPTORS

Insulin receptors are located within the membranes of the cell. When exposed to insulin, a series of events take place that allow glucose to be taken out of the blood vessels and moved into the target cells (liver, muscles, fat cells, etc.).

Because of many factors that include excess glucose and fatty acids, inflammation, and stress, insulin receptors can malfunction. As a result, glucose remains circulating in the blood and doesn't get pulled into the cells. This means that cells don't get the energy they may need and blood sugar levels can increase to dangerous levels.

Elevated levels of blood glucose lead to increased amounts of insulin secreted by the pancreas, which leads to more insulin resistance. The abnormally high amounts of insulin needed to attempt to normalize blood sugar levels has a negative impact on other body tissues and organs, leading to increased fat storage, fatty liver and obesity, polycystic ovarian disease (PCOD), blood vessel thickening and hardening, cancer, sodium retention (which leads to elevated blood pressure), and kidney and brain deterioration, to name only a few.[9, 10, 11, 12, 13]

Interestingly, liver and muscles are the first tissues to become insulin-resistant, while fat cells will still store sugars as fat. This leads to loss of muscle mass and increased weight gain in the form of fatty tissue, and further worsening of insulin resistance. This happens long before diabetes is diagnosed and is why being overweight is a very early sign of diabetes to come.

LIVER

The liver is one of the most important organs in the body that helps to regulate blood sugar. In addition to providing healthy digestive function by producing bile acid filtering all products from digestion and detoxification, the liver plays a central role in regulating systemic metabolism, including protein, carbohydrate, and lipid metabolism. All of these are under close control by a series of hormones secreted from various organs. A healthy liver can store and release glucose in response to insulin as needed to help maintain healthy blood sugar levels. Elevated sugars will get processed by the liver into triglycerides to be stored as fat. This leads to a fatty liver and increased fat throughout the body. Circulating insulin in elevated amounts substantially interferes with the other main functions of the liver and will affect general systemic metabolism.

BRAIN

Glucose is the primary fuel for the brain. High levels of blood sugar and insulin can be damaging to the brain. Research has shown an increase in dementia and Alzheimer's disease in patients with blood sugar impairment. A 2012 study described how insulin resistance is involved in the onset and progression of neurodegenerative diseases such as Alzheimer's disease.

The brain essentially controls almost every function in the body, either directly via nerve signals or indirectly via chemical hormone messengers. As such, the brain sends signals to various organs and glands in the body, many of which work to help to regulate blood sugar. The healthier your brain is, the better job it will do controlling blood sugar.

ADRENAL GLANDS

The adrenal glands have a dramatic effect on blood sugars via several hormones they help produce. The adrenals are small, almond-sized glands that sit one on each of your kidneys. They are instrumental in forming progesterone, estrogen, and testosterone, all of which have a hand in blood sugar levels.

The adrenal gland hormone, cortisol, also has an effect on blood sugar. Many refer to the adrenal glands as the "stress" glands. This is because emotional, chemical, and physical stress; tissue damage; inflammation; and pain cause the adrenal glands to release cortisol. This hormone causes glucose to be released from storage and stimulates production of new glucose, all of which results in increased levels of blood sugar.[14] Any elevation in cortisol will create an elevation in blood sugar. Food allergies or infections will do this because they cause an immune response (inflammation) which then triggers the release of cortisol (anti-inflammatory).

THYROID

Thyroid gland dysfunction will also have an impact on blood sugar. Functional thyroid imbalances are very common in the diabetic population and impact blood sugar. A low-functioning thyroid will lead to a slowed metabolism. A slowed metabolism means that sugar isn't burned efficiently.

Cholesterol and blood levels of insulin will also remain high with low-functioning thyroid. These in turn can contribute to worsening of the pre-diabetes or diabetes.

GASTROINTENSTINAL SYSTEM

The gastrointestinal system is connected to every other system in the body. The majority of your immune cells reside in your gut. If your gut isn't working properly, it can cause a cascade of problems including the inability to absorb nutrients and issues with hormone metabolism, energy production, and toxin elimination.

We commonly find that our diabetic patients are dealing with various bacterial, parasitic, and candida infections, oftentimes without any obvious intestinal symptoms. These infections will disrupt the function on the gut, cause increased inflammation, and ultimately have an effect on blood sugar regulation. We have seen fasting blood sugar drop as much as 40 points just after getting rid of an intestinal infection. Remember, infections cause cortisol to be released, which in turn causes sugar to go up.

IMMUNE SYSTEM

Individual food sensitivities or allergies can also have an effect on your immune system and have an impact on your gut and blood sugar. We perform comprehensive food testing on patients that help us customize nutrition plans. Many are amazed to discover the foods they're reacting to.

Other parts of your body are involved with regulating blood sugar, too, but we aren't here to bore you with anatomy and physiology lessons. We want you to understand that in order to properly treat your condition, all of these areas need to be tested, analyzed, and corrected if they aren't functioning properly.

Other immune issues such as autoimmunity can have direct and indirect impacts on blood sugars. Autoimmunity is where the body's immune system has become dysregulated and the body loses its ability to distinguish between itself and foreign invaders that need to be attacked and destroyed. As a result, your immune system starts to attack and destroy tissues in the body itself. If the pancreas is attacked, this can lead to Type 1 diabetes. Attack on any tissue, because it's inflammation, will indirectly result in sugars being high due to the likely release of cortisol (anti-inflammatory).

1

START WITH THE RIGHT MINDSET

It's easy to be healthy and stay healthy with the right mindset. Well, actually, it's easy to do, and it's easy not to do. Every day we make both healthy and unhealthy choices. The results of these daily decisions aren't always instantly apparent to us. Whenever we feel no immediate discomfort, it becomes very easy to make an unhealthy diet choice.

Consider the following scenario: You're out for dinner with a group of friends and the server asks about dessert. Your conscience tells you to make the healthy decision and decline the super-sized piece of chocolate cake; however, eating the chocolate cake is far more appealing. You know the dessert isn't going to make you healthier and that eating it will push you farther away from your health goals. You think to yourself, "It's only this one dessert, it won't hurt. And besides, everyone else is having dessert, and it's Friday. I've had a long week. I deserve it."

You probably won't notice a difference in your health the next day whether you eat the dessert or not. If you give in and have it, the mindset that fueled the decision to do so will make a significant difference over time—the difference between whether or not you achieve your health goals. Eating the cake justifies the same decision in the future. This exposes a flaw in your mindset. In the short term, your health doesn't appear to be compromised. But in the long term, your health deteriorates many hundreds of times over each time you make a harmful diet choice. The key to good health is to make the right, easy decision consistently and repetitively. To do this, you must develop the right mindset.

The first step toward achieving your health goals is knowing why you have these goals. The health goals of most of our patients include losing weight, reducing medications, having more energy, sleeping better, eating healthier, and so on. These are all terrific goals, but just as New Year's resolutions can be easily forgotten, so, too, can these goals be ignored if the real reasons you want to achieve them aren't uncovered.

Start by writing down your goals. Take out a piece of paper, or better yet, a binder, so you have a place to write notes later. List your goals, then write why they're important to you. Why do you want to lose weight? Why do you want to eat well? Why do you want to be healthy? What will you be able to do once you achieve these goals? What are those key elements in your life that are motivating you to achieve these goals? What are you living for? What are the things that you're passionate about that you want to continue to do? It may be that you want to be around to spend time with your children, grandchildren, or spouse. Whatever the reasons, you need to take the time to figure out what's right for you and write it down. Also write down how it will feel when you achieve these goals. Record all of the many likely sensations you will experience once you achieve your goals. These core motivating factors will determine your long-term success or failure.

It's also essential to remember that there are no shortcuts to becoming healthy. Various health ads and commercials try to entice people to use the next miracle pill or procedure. These shortcuts are usually temporary bandages, not long-term solutions. Many times these shortcuts can make your health worse. It takes motivation and determination, followed by the right decisions and actions, to achieve your health goals. There's no quick fix.

Having the right mindset can make or break your ability to achieve overall health and wellness. Achieving your goals isn't impossible. In fact, as long as your goals are realistic, you can do anything that you set your mind to. If you don't take the time to determine the benefits and advantages of becoming healthy, then you won't have the motivation needed to be successful. By writing down your goals, you're much more likely to stick to the plan. Without a plan, you aren't likely to achieve your personal goals for health and wellness.

WARNING: Don't skip this step. It's your first building block to achieving your health goals. Completing this step could mean the difference between your long-term success and failure.

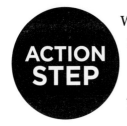

Write down your health goals. Next to those goals, record why you want to achieve each one and why it's important to you. Then write down how you imagine yourself looking, feeling, and acting once you achieve these goals.

2

START YOUR DAY WITH A HIGH-QUALITY BREAKFAST

We've all heard that breakfast is the most important meal of the day. There's a lot of truth in that, but breakfast seems to be the easiest meal to skip. And not surprisingly, there are risks associated with skipping the most important meal of the day. In fact, the consequences are hazardous to your health.

Breakfast gets your metabolism started for the rest of the day. It literally means that you "break" the "fast." When you wake up, your body comes out of an eight-hour sleep cycle during which you fasted. If you don't eat breakfast within an hour of waking up, you're setting your body up for a blood sugar rollercoaster for the entire day. Several recent studies have determined that skipping breakfast causes stress and is associated with an increased prevalence in type 2 diabetes and obesity.[15, 16]

If you find yourself running out of time in the morning, set your alarm clock back just a bit so you won't be so rushed each day. Here are tips for eating a quality breakfast that will help you start your day the right way.

Start with a high-quality protein, healthy fat, and vegetables. (We generally feel that fruit's better as a snack.) It's easy to get many of these ingredients into a breakfast shake. A protein powder, preferably made from rice, pea or collagen protein, is a great shake ingredient. Add 1/4 cup of nuts or 1 tablespoon of nut butter—walnuts, almonds, or almond butter work wonderfully. Add a couple handfuls of leafy greens, celery, cucumber, broccoli, veggie sprouts, and so on (you get the idea). You can also add green vegetable powder or antioxident powders and chia or flax seeds. Blend these ingredients together with some water or almond or coconut milk for a quick and easy breakfast treat. You can also add omega-3 fatty acids to your morning shake, along with any other liquid or powdered vitamins you take. If you are struggling with the flavor, it's also great to add 1 to 2 tablespoons of raw organic cocoa powder.

Protein and fats are the keys to a healthy breakfast. They keep your sugars from spiking to a critical level and help them remain at the right level through the first half of your day.

Other great breakfast choices are turkey bacon (nitrate and gluten-free), chicken, or turkey sausage with a pile of steamed veggies. Honestly, nothing quite beats some leftover rotisserie chicken, steamed broccoli, and olive oil dressing for the most important meal of the day. We recommend this option to all of the diabetics in our office. This leads to our next important tip.

ACTION STEP

Create a grocery list with the items you need to start your day, including a high-quality protein. Figure out what you need to do to prepare and eat your breakfast daily. Do you need to get up a little earlier or prepare food ahead of time so that you can just warm it up? These are just a couple of simple ideas that will help you get started with eating a great breakfast each morning. If you're not used to eating breakfast, then you may find it to be a bit difficult at first. Once you get into a routine, though, you'll find that your new approach isn't hard to follow.

3

EAT ON A SCHEDULE

We know many of you lose track of time and get so caught up with what you're doing that you often completely forget to eat meals or snacks. You keep pushing your meal or snack back later and later as you rush to meet deadlines. While you may think this is no big deal, it's actually quite detrimental to your health, especially if you already have diabetes. Blood sugar swings caused by skipping meals or snacks sets the stage for chronic disease—especially diabetes.[17]

You can combat this problem by making sure you don't go more than two or three hours without eating something. The challenge is to remember to eat something even when you're busy and perhaps not even hungry. Set a reminder on your phone, kitchen timer, or computer. This reminder approach is very effective because we can only consciously focus on one thing at a time, and it's usually not eating until we are super hungry. That's a sign that you've gone too long without food and means you're more likely to over-eat to make up for it. An audible reminder will encourage you to take a break.

Your snacks can be as simple as nuts, veggies and humus or other bean dips, a piece of fruit, trail mix, or a healthy food or protein bar. Many of you will need to eat your fruit with some protein, such as nuts or nut butters, to keep your sugars and insulin surges down. You'll know this is the case if you eat and then find your energy crashes and you become very tired, or if you eat your fruit and become hungry right after doing so. Stick to only one fruit snack per day and eat it in the morning. This gives you a chance to burn the sugar as fuel during the most active part of the day while it helps you avoid sugars spikes at night.

We know you're thinking that you're going to gain weight by doing this, but just the opposite will occur: You will lose weight. The key is to provide your body with the right fuel and smaller amounts of carbohydrates and calories at steady intervals. This means staying away from processed foods and eating whole foods every two to three hours.

Your body is a machine that needs the right fuel to function properly. Are you fueling a supercharged sports car or a broken down jalopy? Are you using high-octane fuel or low-grade fuel? Are you pit-stopping often enough during the day to handle the demands of modern life? The food you eat needs to provide your cells, muscles, organs, and tissues with energy. Many of us are in a routine of having breakfast, lunch, and dinner without any thought as to how the food is going to fuel our body. The food we eat affects our performance at work, sleep cycles, moods, family interactions, participation in recreational or physical activities, and ultimately how we will live and die. So think of your food as your fuel and ask yourself if the food you're about to eat will increase or decrease your horsepower.

More and more, food in our society has become a source of entertainment rather than a necessity for function and survival. It needs to look, smell, and taste pretty for people to consider eating it. Eating isn't for entertainment; it's for survival. Knowing what and how to eat will help the food taste great and help you feel great and function well, too.

What's the big deal about eating healthy foods at specific intervals, you ask? Well, when you go too long (more than three hours) without eating so you can fuel your body, your blood sugar begins to drop. One of the main fuels for the brain is glucose. So, as your blood sugar drops, your brain begins to suffer and sends stress signals to your body to get the sugar up. If you fail to eat, the brain triggers the adrenal glands to spit out cortisol, which stimulates the release of sugar from the liver into the blood stream as a response to the stress of blood sugar getting too low.[18, 19]

If this happens daily, it leads to further insulin resistance over time due to the fact that elevated cortisol causes insulin receptors to "shut down" and degrade.[20] By the time you finally get around to eating something, your sugar might already be rising because of the stress of having dropped too low earlier. When you finally eat, the food causes a further boost in your blood sugar, leading to your blood sugar level likely being too high.

Too much sugar is toxic to the body tissues and brain, so your body now has to scramble to pump out lots of insulin from your pancreas to get all this excess sugar out of the blood and into other tissues.[19] Years of this up and down sugar roller coaster leads to insulin resistance, obesity, diabetes, and heart disease. And all of this is partly because you neglected to take five minutes to eat a small snack or to keep to a regular meal schedule. When you did finally eat, you were so hungry you ate the wrong foods, and way too much of them.

Plan your schedule for the typical day. This schedule includes when you wake; eat breakfast, lunch, and dinner; snack in between meals; and go to bed. Use the following chart as an example to help plan your day. Then, find a way to stick to it, no matter what.

Wake Up	Breakfast	Snack	Lunch	Snack	Dinner	Bedtime
6:30 a.m.	7 a.m.	10 a.m.	12:30 p.m.	3:30 p.m.	6:30 p.m.	10:30 p.m.

ACTION STEP

Plan your day to include regularly scheduled meals and snacks. If you have a busy schedule, look for foods you can snack on while you're on the go. Healthy snacks are an important part of balanced nutrition. Snacks that are low in carbohydrates and sugar are the best choices. Useful tip: If you have a difficult time remembering to eat on time, set reminders on your phone or computer at work to help keep yourself on track.

4

GET A GOOD NIGHT'S SLEEP

Our bodies repair, rebuild, and regenerate all of our systems and tissues while we sleep. Sleeping for seven to eight hours may be one of the most important strategies for staying healthy and reducing the chance of developing chronic diseases. If sleeping that long isn't realistic for you now, start making small changes to begin moving in that direction. If you're accustomed to getting only a few hours of sleep, you might want to start by going to bed a bit earlier each night until you're used to the new schedule. This will help ensure that you get an adequate amount of sleep every day.

Running around all day causes plenty of wear on the body. It's essential to get adequate sleep to recharge the body and rebuild worn tissues. Sufficient rest is especially vital for rebuilding bones, recharging the immune system, and keeping diabetes-causing inflammation down.[21,22] One recently published study showed that middle-aged women with shortened sleep cycles are susceptible to metabolic syndrome, the precursor to type 2 diabetes.[23] Another study revealed that young, lean adults with a family history of type 2 diabetes develop insulin resistance and elevated blood insulin levels due to not enough sleep (less than six hours).[24]

If it's a challenge for you to get to bed early, start by moving the television out of the bedroom. Instead of watching television in bed, read before you go to sleep. If possible, move all other electronic devices out of the bedroom—tablets, laptop computers, smartphones, etc. We should be winding down after dinner and before bed, not revving up with stress and anxiety by taking on new projects, finishing work, or watching horror stories on the news.

Exposure to bright lights, such as those from a TV or computer monitor, can prevent your brain from secreting melatonin, the hormone that helps induce a deep, restful sleep. You're more likely to stay up later, be wired, and have a difficult time getting to sleep, or staying asleep, if you're exposing yourself to bright light right before bed.

Plan your ideal sleep schedule, including the specific times you will go to sleep and wake up. Now create the environment to support this ideal schedule. Your sleep rhythms aren't going to change overnight, so be patient and stick to your schedule.

Consider your sleep quality, too. While you may feel like you're getting enough sleep, if you wake up feeling like you didn't really rest well, then you may not be getting high-quality sleep. The quality of your sleep is affected by many different factors. Sometimes lights or other noise in the room can affect your sleep patterns.

If you feel that you're not getting quality sleep on a regular basis—and you aren't quite sure why—you may want to discuss this with your doctor. You might need to go in for a sleep study to see what's going on. Perhaps you're waking up throughout the night without realizing it—that can really hinder your ability to feel well-rested the next day. This can be caused by hormone imbalances (estrogen or progesterone deficiency), glandular insufficiencies (adrenals), brain and neurotransmitter imbalances, infections, or sleep apnea. You want someone who specializes in functional medicine to check for all of them and treat any conditions found.

Sleep isn't important for just those who have diabetes and pre-diabetes. Everyone benefits from getting a good night of sleep.

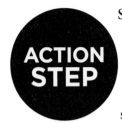

Set a bedtime that targets eight hours of sleep and stick to it. Straying from your sleep schedule from time to time isn't going to throw you completely off, but you should definitely keep to the schedule. Start a nightly routine that will prepare your body for sleep. If you have difficulty going to sleep at night, try a few relaxation techniques such as taking a calming bath before bedtime. Remove electronic gadgets, including a TV, laptop, tablet, and phone to reduce sleep interference.

5

STOP COUNTING CALORIES AND FOLLOW DR. STEPH'S PLATE RULE©

When you sit down for breakfast, lunch, or dinner, how do you know if you have healthy food on your plate? Whether you're eating at home or dining out, the answer to this is actually quite simple. There's no need for complicated formulas, calorie counts, or point systems. What you're eating is more important than how much you're eating if you follow "Dr. Steph's Plate Rule©."

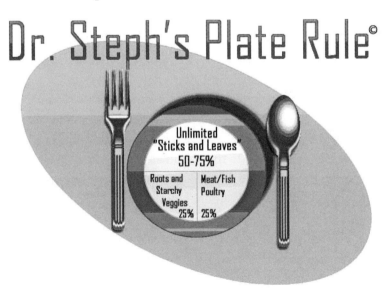

Dr. Steph's Plate Rule©

Unlimited "Sticks and Leaves" 50-75%

Roots and Starchy Veggies 25%

Meat/Fish Poultry 25%

35

One-quarter of your plate should consist of good quality animal protein (3 to 6 ounces). This includes wild-caught fish, grass-fed beef, free-range poultry, or lamb. Another quarter of the plate should consist of up to one-half of a cup of a starchy vegetable, usually a type of root vegetable, such as beets, carrots, sweet potatoes, turnips, squash, etc. Avocado would also fit here. On the remaining half of the plate, put unlimited amounts of vegetables. These include your "sticks and leaves," such as broccoli, peppers, greens, lettuce, spinach, and so on.

Over the top of the entire plate (or just on your vegetables), pour a home-made dressing made from a simple recipe of extra virgin cold-pressed organic olive oil, freshly crushed garlic, dried or fresh green herbs, lemon juice or vinegar (raw cider, organic balsamic, etc.)—see page 108 for the recipe. Dr. Steph recommends keeping a bottle of this on-hand and ready to go for easy use. Fat is very important because it helps you digest and absorb more nutrients from your vegetables than you would get without fat, and it also helps you feel full and happy after eating your meal. When you eat this way, you will feel satisfied and not have the cravings associated with a high sugar/high carbohydrate meal.

Shopping at your local produce stand is a great way to get started. You will want to make sure you keep a large stock of leafy vegetables that are great for filling you up at mealtime. If your plate looks full, you will be less likely to overindulge in other things that aren't as great for your health. If you follow the plate rule and fill at least half of your plate with vegetables, then you will likely find yourself not going back for seconds at mealtime. If you do decide that you want to go back for a second helping, just get a second helping of the veggies instead of the starchy foods and meat. This will help to promote a much healthier diet and lead to better nutrition, which is essential to those who are diabetic or pre-diabetic.

Fruits, beans, nuts, and limited grains are best eaten for snacks. When it comes to fruits, they should be eaten in moderation (one to two per day max), especially if working to reverse your diabetes. While they are a healthy and important part of your daily nutrition, they are also full of natural sugars. These sugars can raise your blood glucose levels and worsen insulin resistance. As long as you eat fruits in moderation, however, they shouldn't be harmful to your blood glucose levels. Choose organic fruits because they will have fewer additives and harmful chemicals. The best place to find organic fruit is your local farmer's market or produce stand. Most non-organic fruits in your chain grocery store have been treated with chemicals and other additives.

ACTION STEP

Before you fix your plate at mealtime, make sure that you remember the "plate rule." This is for all meals, including breakfast. You can do this easily by printing out the graphic above and placing it somewhere highly visible, such as on your refrigerator door. Take a look at it before you put your food on your plate, and then make sure that you stick to it. It should only take two weeks before it becomes a natural habit and you will no longer need the picture's guidance. See APPENDIX A for a list of foods put into categories to help you build your meal and snack plates.

The plate rule meal can be consumed in the form of a meal shake, which many people prefer for breakfast, especially during the busy work week. With a blender such as a Nutrabullet, Ninja, or Vitamix, blend a high quality protein powder, 1 or more cups of "sticks and leaves" veggies, 1 tablespoon of olive oil or coconut oil, and 1 tablespoon of chia or flax seeds with as much water as you need to get the consistency you like. If you feel you can't drink this without some fruit, keep frozen berries or banana chunks on hand and pop a few into the shake. You don't want to consume a fruit smoothie with a pile of fruit in it for breakfast—this will spike your sugars and you'll be very hungry by mid-morning.

SHOP THE OUTER AISLES OF THE GROCERY STORE

The easiest way to stay away from processed foods is by shopping in the outer aisles of the grocery store.

Think about the layout of your local supermarket. You will likely find that the majority of the staples you need for a balanced diet are found on the store's perimeter—the outer aisles. For instance, milk, bread, meat, and produce ring the center of the grocery store. The majority of the foods you find on those inner aisles are cookies, crackers, snack cakes, ice cream, and a lot of other processed foods that are full of sugar and other additives.

In the outer aisles, you'll find fruits, vegetables, and proteins. These are the foods you want on your plate. You may need to venture down a couple of aisles to get oils, condiments, seasoning, or snacks. Just make sure you're reading labels and avoiding any processed groceries. Most of the center aisles are filled with chemical-laden foods that contribute to chronic disease.

If you shop the outer aisles, you will definitely save a lot of time and money while you find that you have a much healthier diet. But note that one of the biggest mistakes you can make is going to the grocery store without a list and then wandering up and down each aisle picking things up just because they look good. Without a list or a plan, you will likely go home with far too many unnecessary items, and only a few truly nutritious foods.

ACTION STEP

If you have a tendency to buy a lot of processed foods, you may want to make a grocery list and vow to stick to it. When you're making that list, start by visualizing your local supermarket and listing the items as you would find them in the store. This will help keep you out of the middle aisles as much as possible. Plan your week's meals ahead of time, too. Then you'll know exactly what you need to get and how the items will combine.

Also, get in the habit of reading all labels before placing items in your cart. Once you get used to shopping smart, you should be able to recognize the items that are healthy without having to read every label.

7

BUY GRASS-FED BEEF AND MEATS

You're probably surprised that we're recommending eating beef at all. That's because not all beef is created equal. The old saying, "You are what you eat" also applies to the animals you eat. There are grass-fed cows and there are grain-fed cows. Grass-fed cattle are healthy and a great source of disease-preventing protein and fat. The meat from grain-fed cattle is fattier and contains higher amounts of inflammation-causing fats than meat from grass-fed cattle.[25] We're pretty certain that if they were permitted to live longer, grain-fed cattle would likely become obese and diabetic, just as humans do on similar diets.

Cattle are designed to eat grass, but the farming industry has evolved such that farmers feed cattle grain to fatten them up and marbleize their meat before slaughter. Farmers who use grain feed are able to grow and confine more cattle per square foot of land. That provides a greater yield, which equals bigger profits and savings. The bigger the animal, the more beef it supplies, and the more money per cow is made. Sounds good, right?

Wrong.

Grain-fed cattle yield a different type of beef. Our bodies metabolize it differently than grass-fed beef. A grass-fed cow has a stomach pH of 7; its grain-fed counterpart's is 4. This acidic pH of 4, along with the different fat composition of the food itself, impedes the production of healthy fats like conjugated linoleic acid (CLA) and omega-3, and increases the production of omega-6 fatty acids.[25] A diet rich in CLA has been shown to have a positive effect on glycemic control, increase insulin sensitivity, and have the potential to help prevent diabetes.[26, 27]

Michael Pollan, author, wrote in The *New York Times* about what happens to cows when they're taken off of pastures, put into feedlots, and fed grain:

"Perhaps the most serious thing that can go wrong with a ruminant on corn is feedlot bloat. The rumen is always producing copious amounts of gas, which is normally expelled by belching during rumination. But when the diet contains too much starch and too little roughage, rumination all but stops, and a layer of foamy slime that can trap gas forms in the rumen. The rumen inflates like a balloon, pressing against the animal's lungs. Unless action is promptly taken to relieve the pressure (usually by forcing a hose down the animal's esophagus), the cow suffocates.

"A corn diet can also give a cow acidosis. Unlike that in our own highly acidic stomachs, the normal pH of a rumen is neutral. Corn makes it unnaturally acidic, however, causing a kind of bovine heartburn, which in some cases can kill the animal but usually just makes it sick. Acidotic animals go off their feed, pant and salivate excessively, paw at their bellies and eat dirt. The condition can lead to diarrhea, ulcers, bloat, liver disease, and a general weakening of the immune system that leaves the animal vulnerable to everything from pneumonia to feedlot polio."

The average American diet already consists of an excess of inflammation-causing omega-6 fats and not enough inflammation-lowering omega-3 fats. Consuming grain-fed beef further contributes to this unhealthy fat ratio. The fact that corn is the main grain eaten by cattle is a particular concern because corn is full of omega 6 inflammatory fats, so it further exacerbates anyone's already poor diet.

So, how do you know whether or not the beef that you're purchasing is from cows that have been grass- or grain-fed? Check the labels, since supermarket beef is labeled as to whether or not it's grass-fed. If you're buying from a local meat market, you may need to talk to the manager to get the information you need.

Now that you're aware of the difference between grass-fed and grain-fed beef, you can make smarter choices. When eating out, it's sometimes difficult to ensure that you're eating grass-fed beef. Discuss this with the chef before ordering. If the chef is unsure, then chances are they aren't serving grass-fed beef. At home, you can use grass-fed beef for any recipe that calls for beef.

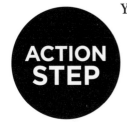

You don't have to steer clear of beef altogether. Instead, make sure that you check labels to ensure that the beef you're purchasing has been grass-fed. It will always say so on the package. If you shop at a local meat market, ask the manager to help you with your selection. Look for grass-fed beef at local farmers markets or co-ops, too.

8

EAT WILD-CAUGHT FISH

Did you know that some of the fish you buy is caught wild and some of it is farm-raised? Farm-raised fish may sound good, but it's usually treated with coloring, antibiotics, and other medications.[28] These treatments prevent infections caused by overcrowding. Wild-caught fish, on the other hand, are able to swim freely in their natural habitat, eating foods they were meant to eat. They are healthy and provide the nutrients your body needs to be healthy, too.

The primary nutrients you get from wild-caught fish, other than protein, are the omega-3 fatty acids, especially from salmon. These are the good fats that you need for proper nerve, brain, cell, organ, and tissue function. Omega-3 fats also contribute to heart and artery health, balancing cholesterol, and reducing inflammation. Farm-raised fish have hardly any of these good fats and are full of chemicals that can prevent you from actually getting the nutrients that fish is known for. That means that you're basically choosing fish as a healthier option, but you're avoiding the healthy advantages if you're not selecting wild-caught fish.

When dining out, ask about the source. If it's farm-raised, take a pass on it. For home consumption, look for stores that sell wild-caught fish. You want to make sure that the fish you're choosing is actually good for you. Several stores, including wholesale clubs such as Costco and Sam's Club, sell wild fish in their frozen seafood section. Interestingly, it was at one of these stores a few years ago that we first discovered that coloring was added to the farm-raised fish. You can also find great wild-caught fish at your local seafood market. Ask the manager for help identifying which is wild-caught and which is farm-raised. You might be surprised to find out what they have to offer.

Your options for finding wild-caught fish don't stop there. You can also find sources online; Vital Choice will ship several types of frozen wild fish right to your door—all in a sustainable fashion. It doesn't get more convenient than that.

ACTION STEP

When you want to buy fish, avoid shopping at the last minute. If you shop for fish ahead of time, you can get the wild-caught fish you need. Shopping online is a great option, especially if you like to eat fish a few times a week. The fish is conveniently frozen so all you need to do is thaw and prepare it. If you're shopping in your local supermarket, be sure to read the labels. We can't stress this enough.

9

EAT ORGANIC FREE-RANGE POULTRY

Most of us eat poultry in the form of turkey and chicken. You want to eat organic free-range poultry for the same reason you want to eat grass-fed beef: Research shows that organic free-range poultry has higher levels of omega-3 fatty acids, conjugated linoleic acids (CLA), and beta-carotene.[29] An Iowa State University study showed that organic free-range chickens have higher levels of protein when compared to conventional birds. Organic free-range poultry is also less likely to be diseased and contain hormones, antibiotics, and other additives.[30] In addition, studies have shown that non-organic poultry can have a negative impact on your health.

What exactly is free-range poultry? The U.S. Department of Agriculture defines it as poultry that's allowed to have access to outside areas. Basically, these animals aren't kept in cages and are allowed to roam free outside during the day. Be careful when choosing your organic free-range poultry, though, because even chickens and turkeys that are allowed outside for just a short period of time may be marked "free-range." The best way to ensure that you're getting genuine free-range poultry is to buy it from a local farmer who guarantees it. Ensure that the poultry roamed a pasture for the majority of the day and that the grass was pesticide-free.

Note, too, that free-range poultry and organic free-range poultry are two different things. Just because poultry is free-range doesn't necessarily mean that it's organic. Organic poultry isn't treated with the chemicals and other additives—antibiotics and growth hormones—that other poultry receives. The USDA National Organic Program enforces certain standards regarding all organic foods, meats, and produce that all farmers must comply with. When shopping in your local grocery store, look for the brown and green "USDA Organic" seal before purchasing the poultry. This seal indicates that the poultry is at least 95 percent organic.

Look for organic free-range poultry in your grocery store or find a local farmer to buy from. While the number of small farms is on the decline, you can probably still find a few within a certain radius of your home. The smaller poultry farmers generally raise their poultry in a natural setting and they pay close attention to quality. They are also concerned with the well being of their animals. That means that you'll often find local free-range poultry that is also organic. If you have a hard time finding a local farmer with these options, check your local health food store, since they often offer locally raised poultry. Chances are they will be able to point you in the right direction.

ACTION STEP

Avoid buying poultry that has been treated with hormones and other additives. If you're unsure about the poultry you normally buy, read the label. Sometimes the best way to ensure that you're getting poultry that is free of additives is to buy locally from a farmer. While you may spend a bit more on organic free-range poultry, it's a good investment for your health.

10

CHECK YOUR VITAMIN D LEVEL AND GET IT OPTIMIZED

The majority of our patients lack vitamin D–deplorably so. Vitamin D is critical for functions such as preventing cancer, osteoporosis, type 1 and type 2 diabetes, and heart disease. It also contributes to healthy pancreas function and insulin sensitivity and maintaining healthy brain function.[26, 31, 32, 33, 34, 35, 36]

JoEllen Welsh, a researcher with the State University of New York at Albany, has studied vitamin D for more than two decades. In a 2010 interview with the *ABC Network,* she reported that in one of her research studies on breast cancer, large doses of vitamin D destroyed 50 percent of the cancer cells.[37] It stands to reason that if we optimize our vitamin D levels as an entire population, we might be able to reduce the incidence of cancer significantly. This statement may sound overly optimistic, but it's being supported by more and more published research.

Our bodies naturally produce vitamin D while exposed to the sun. There was a time in history when people worked outside most of the day from spring until fall, so their bodies produced vitamin D naturally in high levels, stockpiling it for the winter months. Unfortunately, modern times have led us primarily indoors, where most of us sit at a computer under florescent lights. As a result, many of us don't get enough sun exposure to maintain optimal vitamin D levels.

The range for optimal functional blood levels of vitamin D are from

40-100 ng/ml with the ideal range—especially if you have cancer or diabetes—being 80 ng/ml.[38] We target our patients' levels for at least above 60 ng/ml. If you don't know your level, ask your doctor to check when you go in for your next blood test. If you find that you're low, include a vitamin D3 supplement in your diet. It may require up to 10,000 i.u.s per day or more to get your levels up to between 60-80 ng/ml. The only way to know is to get tested and then follow up in a few months to see where you are. You can purchase a vitamin D3 supplement over the counter. Surprisingly, this is one of the cheapest supplements you can find. Often, prescription vitamin D will be in the form D2, but this isn't the ideal form. Look for D3.

You can also boost your vitamin D production naturally. After all, the majority of your vitamin D is stored in your body during the spring and summer months so that you don't have a deficiency during the winter. Your liver stores vitamin D for the winter months so if your liver is in good condition, it can store up to four months' worth. This is important because most people don't spend a lot of time outdoors in the sun during the winter. While the sun is the best way to receive your vitamin D naturally, there are other options, including:

- Eating bitter foods or herbs to help stimulate bile, which is important when it comes to vitamin D absorption and production.
- Eating spices that are helpful to your digestive system.
- Adding mushrooms to your diet because they help produce vitamin D.

There are a few common misconceptions when it comes to vitamin D. First, many people think that it's a vitamin—for obvious reasons—but it's not. Just like a peanut isn't a nut but rather a legume, vitamin D isn't so much a vitamin as it is a hormone, one that is produced naturally by the body. More specifically, it's secosteroid hormone. This is a bit different than other steroids, such as testosterone, cholesterol, and cortisol.

Another misconception is that vitamin D supplements are all that you need. These supplements still require adequate amounts of sunlight, pancreatic enzymes, and intestinal proteins in order to be effective. So if you're taking D3 supplements, make sure that you're getting the most out of them in order to get the full benefits from adequate levels of vitamin D.

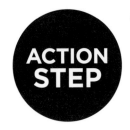

Ask your physician to test your vitamin D levels. A simple blood test provides your current levels. If they aren't where they need to be (we target our patients to blood levels of 60-80 ng/ml), add a vitamin D 3 supplement. Once you have been on the supplement for a few months, schedule another visit with your doctor and have your vitamin D levels rechecked.

More importantly, look for ways to stimulate your body's vitamin D production naturally. Get outside at least 30 to 60 minutes each day during the warmer spring and summer months so you get direct sunlight on your skin. We don't want you to burn, so avoid peak times of the day and start in the spring with only a few minutes at a time to build up tolerance. This is the best source of vitamin D for your body and offers the most health benefits. If that's not possible based on your job schedule or where you live, you can buy a tanning bed that emits the UV light needed by your body to make vitamin D. They can be expensive, so you'll want to shop around if you decide to do this.

11

EAT FRESH, ORGANIC, NON-GMO FRUITS AND VEGETABLES

Fruits and vegetables are an important part of your diet. If you're eating mainly canned or frozen vegetables, we encourage you to start eating fresh, organic vegetables. When that isn't possible, organic frozen is better than none at all. Remember, when you're following Dr. Steph's Plate Rule©, you will be eating large portions of vegetables (50 to 75 percent of all of your meals), so you want these to be the best quality possible.

Many consumers now believe that organic is more nutritious then conventional. Is this fact or just clever marketing? Organic is best mainly because you're limiting your exposure to the highly toxic pesticides, herbicides, and other chemicals that are sprayed on non-organic produce. Organic foods also have a higher level of nutrients such as iron, vitamin C, phosphorus, and magnesium when compared to non-organic foods.[39]

In recent decades, we've also seen a huge rise in genetically modified organisms (GMO), which in many instances means the plant's DNA has been altered so that it includes the pesticide or herbicide, or it's been designed genetically to produce that pesticide or herbicide. It could also be genetically modified to tolerate sprayed herbicides so the weeds die, but the crop doesn't. In that situation, farmers often use more herbicides than usual to kill the weeds because the GMO crop can survive the onslaught. This translates to more herbicides in our diet when we consume GMO foods.

The higher amounts of chemicals sprayed (ironic since we were "sold" on the idea that GMOs would mean fewer chemicals) has led to increased resistance for weeds and insects, creating "super weeds." As a result, farmers need to spray even more chemicals than before to grow their crops. The GMO acronym essentially means that even washing the food won't eliminate the poisons because they're part of the plant.

When you can't find organic vegetables and fruits, choose non-organic produce that requires peeling before eating and, if possible, produce that is non-GMO. This minimizes the amount of chemicals you will consume. Berries, lettuce, and spinach should always be organic—there is no way you're peeling and scrubbing each blueberry or lettuce leaf before you eat it. The Environmental Working Group has put out a list of "Dirty Dozen'" foods that must be organic and a list of the "Clean Fifteen," foods that have the least amount of chemicals on them. This is good to have on hand when you may be challenged to find fruits and veggies out of season or when you need to be more careful with your budget.

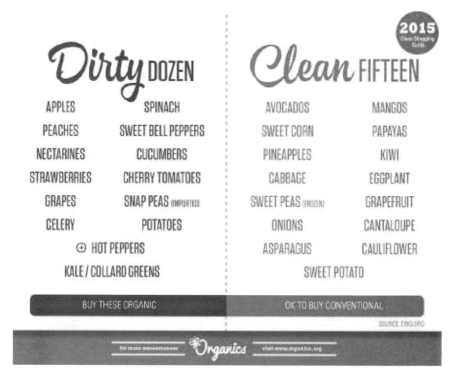

Dirty DOZEN	
APPLES	SPINACH
PEACHES	SWEET BELL PEPPERS
NECTARINES	CUCUMBERS
STRAWBERRIES	CHERRY TOMATOES
GRAPES	SNAP PEAS (IMPORTED)
CELERY	POTATOES
⊕ HOT PEPPERS	
KALE / COLLARD GREENS	

BUY THESE ORGANIC

Clean FIFTEEN	
AVOCADOS	MANGOS
SWEET CORN	PAPAYAS
PINEAPPLES	KIWI
CABBAGE	EGGPLANT
SWEET PEAS (FROZEN)	GRAPEFRUIT
ONIONS	CANTALOUPE
ASPARAGUS	CAULIFLOWER
SWEET POTATO	

OK TO BUY CONVENTIONAL

2015
Clean Shopping Guide

SOURCE: EWG.ORG

Organics

So why are pesticides and herbicides so bad? Generally, these chemicals have been linked to many severe health issues. Some can have long-term consequences and may dramatically shorten lifespan. Studies have shown that these chemicals can cause respiratory issues, celiac disease, infertility, problems with your skin, neurological problems, and even cancer.[40, 41] In fact, in a formal paper dated March 20, 2015, the World Health Organization's International Agency for Research on Cancer, after evaluating five organophosphate insecticides and herbicides, stated that "the herbicide glyphosate and the insecticides malathion and diazinon were classified as probably carcinogenic to humans."

There's even more to eating organic than trying to avoid the chemicals. Organic fruits and veggies offer higher amounts of many of the essential vitamins and minerals that your body needs when those products are grown in organic soil. Organic crop soils are generally much more mineral- and nutrient-rich. When you get these vitamins and minerals naturally from foods with all of the other cofactors and compounds within the food, the body does a better job of absorbing and utilizing them. While you can always take supplements to help you get more of them, your body won't fully absorb and use them like it does with the vitamins and minerals that you get naturally. Those are consumed in concert with hundreds of other natural substances such as other antioxidants, bioflavonoids, plant sterols, etc.

Organic fruits and vegetables also taste better. The fact that there are no chemicals and additives helps them retain their natural flavor. So, not only is organic better for you, but your taste buds will thank you as well. (Do you even remember what tomatoes used to taste like?)

When you buy locally whether it's at the farmer's market or directly from the farm, you often spend less, too. After all, you're not paying the costs associated with shipping from other states or countries.

You can also save a lot more money by starting your own organic garden. It's an interesting hobby that also boosts your overall health and wellness—if you have a place to do it. Even if you don't have much room, a small organic herb garden can really boost the nutrient value of the meals you use them in.

Remember: 75 percent of the foods you eat throughout the day should be vegetables.

ACTION STEPS

1. **Donate any canned fruits and vegetables that you may have in your pantry.** Don't buy them again.

2. **Buy fresh, organic, fruits and vegetables whenever possible.** You can do this at a local grocery store or farmer's market. Talk to the farmer at the market to make sure you're getting organic produce. Print out the Dirty Dozen/Clean Fifteen lists (or take a picture with your phone) to reference when you shop. Consider growing your own fruits and vegetables, too.

3. **Stock up on fruits and vegetables to eat as snacks each day.** Sorting them into small snack bags makes it easier to make smart choices at snack time.

4. **Learn different ways to cook and prepare your vegetables:** Steam, sautee, roast, grill, pressure cook, boil and mash, blend into shakes, eat raw for salads and snacks, use in soups, and so on.

5. **Get lots of variety.** If you haven't been much of a vegetable eater and you've been living on green beans and corn most of your life, buy a new vegetable each week. Look up recipes online or in your favorite cookbook and experiment. Don't buy the ones you don't like again (or look for new recipes) and add the vegetables you like to your regular rotation on your grocery list.

12

GO GRAIN-FREE THEN STAY GLUTEN-FREE

There has been a lot of press given to gluten recently, and rightfully so. Gluten is a protein found primarily in wheat, and also in rye, barley, and spelt. It can be cross-contaminated into other grains, such as oats. Kenneth Fine, M.D., Gastroenterologist and founder of EnteroLab, estimates that 81 percent of the population has a genetic predisposition to gluten reactivity, whether they're displaying symptoms or not. We see more positive test results for this on initial testing with patients in our office than with anything else except for vitamin D deficiency.

Symptoms indicating a possible issue with gluten could include diarrhea, bloating, gas, fatigue, brain fog, joint pain, and inflammation. But you don't have to display symptoms for it to have a negative effect on your body and health. Long-term consumption of gluten has been linked to celiac disease, diabetes,[42] autoimmune thyroiditis (Hashimoto's disease) and other autoimmune diseases, osteoporosis, cardiovascular disease, and neurodegenerative diseases such as Parkinson's, multiple sclerosis, and Alzheimer's. Why tempt fate with this one?

There are tests available to determine if you're reacting to gluten or any of the associated wheat breakdown products. These specialized tests aren't usually performed in the conventional model of health care. One way to see if there is a possibility that you're reacting is to cut gluten-containing foods from your diet for a 30 to 60 day period. During this period, pay attention to how you feel and function (energy levels, bowel movements, and aches and pains). The changes may be subtle, so pay close attention.

However, you must have gluten in your diet if you're going to be tested for gluten intolerance or celiac disease through laboratory testing. If you have been on a gluten-free diet for weeks or months before testing, results may not be accurate. The removal of gluten, or any food that your immune system reacts to, allows the immune system to calm down and stop reacting. Testing for heightened immune markers to gluten after gluten has been removed may give 'false negatives', meaning the immune markers may no longer be present, not because you're not 'reactive', but simply because the trigger has not been present to cause a reaction.

The more we study the research on gluten's impact, the more we believe that everyone should permanently eliminate it from their diets to reduce the likelihood of being diagnosed with a chronic disease. It's easy to go gluten-free. Most supermarkets have a growing selection of gluten-free options, as do many restaurants. We distribute many tasty gluten-free recipes to our patients. Patients enjoy these recipes and soon learn how to devise their own. Check out our book *Lose the Gluten, Lose Your Gut. Ditch the Grain, Save Your Brain* for a complete guide to gluten and living gluten-free.

There are a variety of different benefits that come from a gluten-free diet other than just reducing your risk of type 2 diabetes. First of all, you will find that it removes a lot of pressure on your digestive system. You may not realize it, but wheat is one of the most difficult foods to digest. This can sometimes cause you to have stomach issues such as gas, cramps, and diarrhea. When you start eating gluten-free, you may have far fewer digestive issues.

Another great benefit of removing gluten is the fact that it can help you lose weight. After all, gluten is responsible for a lot of water retention and bloating. This is uncomfortable, but it can also cause you to see a much higher number on the scale. Losing weight is great if you're diabetic or pre-diabetic.

You can also find dermatological benefits when you cut gluten out of your diet. Studies show that people who eat less food with gluten have a clearer complexion. So, while you're working on a healthier gluten-free diet, you can also improve the look of your skin.

Let's discuss grain in general. When we work with patients to reverse their diabetes, we always have them cut out all grains from their diet initially, not just those with gluten. This is for several reasons:

1. Grains contain carbohydrates that convert to sugar
    in your body.
2. Grains contain higher amounts of inflaming fats
    (Omega 6 versus Omega 3).
3. When consuming gluten-free grains, many people have
    immune reactions that are similar to a gluten reaction.
    These reactions cause their immune systems to attack those
    foods as though they contained gluten. That, in turn, can
    lead to prolonged elevations in blood sugar.
4. Most grain products are processed so much that they are
    high-glycemic foods. That means that they will be more
    likely to cause fast and high blood sugar spikes than foods
    that are less processed are more low-glycemic.

As long as your sugars are high and you're working to reverse your diabetes and get sugars into a low range, we suggest you cut out all grains. Once you've reversed your diabetes, we encourage you to stay grain-free, but if you need or want to eat them from time to time, stick with those that are gluten-free to keep inflammation down. There is evidence that shows that gluten reactivity can lead to the immune system's destruction of your pancreas. That can cause a type 2 diabetic who has a genetic pre-disposition to autoimmunity to also become an insulin-dependent type 1 diabetic.[43]

Gluten-free grains include rice, corn (no, corn isn't a vegetable), millet, amaranth, buckwheat, and sorghum. Hemp and quinoa, although they aren't grains, are seeds that are often cooked and eaten as grains. They are higher in protein and generally less inflaming, which can help keep you diabetes-free once you've gotten there.

We recommend that if you insist on eating grain, eat only from the list of gluten-free grains, and in limited quantities (no more that 1 to 2 times per day at 1/2 cup max). It's ideal that you avoid grains altogether, at least until your diabetes is reversed and your sugars are maintained in normal range. Grains such as rice and corn are very high in carbohydrates, which ultimately become sugar in the body.

To avoid gluten, especially when it's medically necessary, read labels of commercially made products such as spice mixes, soups, sauces, broths, and even processed meat products, which can contain gluten for added flavor or binding properties (think "meat glue").

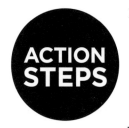

1. **Initially, until sugars are in normal range, cut grains out completely.**

2. **Once your sugars and HbA1c are down in normal range and you're off most or all of your diabetes medications, then you may try, in small amounts, some gluten-free grain products.** Limit this to 1 to 2 servings per day to remain diabetes-free. Consume it without other starches or fats.

3. **Follow a gluten-free diet for the rest of your life.** While it may not be the easiest diet out there for beginners, you can find recipes online that are both delicious and nutritious. Any paleo recipes will be grain-, gluten-, and dairy-free. Check the health food section in your local grocery store for gluten-free items to keep in your pantry. Start by eliminating the gluten from your diet a little bit at a time, and as time goes on, it will become much easier for you to have a completely gluten-free diet.

4. **Grains and foods that are touted as "whole grain" can often contain more sugar or sugar potential than candy.** You should have already eliminated grains to reverse diabetes, and you will be very cautious when bringing them back into your diet by sticking primarily to gluten-free products. A word of caution about bringing back even gluten-free grains: Gluten-free grain products are also manufactured with and contain significant amounts of sugar, so watch out. While reversing your diabetes, try eliminating grains completely (following Dr. Steph's Plate Rule©). Once reversed and re-introducing gluten-free grains, limit them to no more than 1 to 2 servings per day at 1/2 cup maximum.

13

REDUCE OR ELIMINATE SUGAR INTAKE

Research estimates that the average American consumes 22 teaspoons of sugar per day.[44] Sugar can be difficult to detect when it's disguised and hidden in the ingredient lists under various names on processed food packaging. It's most often listed under other more scientifically specific chemical and technical names. The majority of processed foods contain different sugars with names such as "high fructose corn syrup" and "dextrose." Whether it's white table sugar or sugar identified with one of these disguised scientific names, it must be minimized for overall health and virtually eliminated while working to reverse your diabetes. Sugar cause a rise in insulin levels and ultimately worsens diabetes, inhibits hormone production, depresses the immune system, causes weight gain, cardiovascular dysfunction, cancer, Alzheimer's disease, dental decay, and an overall shortening of lifespan.[45, 46, 47, 48]

When you're diabetic, dramatically reducing sugar intake is critical. If you don't commit to this step, you will not reverse diabetes. Type 2 diabetes is caused by a sugar overload relative to your body's insulin receptor sensitivity and the amount of circulating insulin. When you eat foods that have a lot of sugar, your blood sugar will rise. To lower that blood sugar, the pancreas secretes insulin. If you don't have the ability to make enough insulin to handle the sugars, or if your cells' insulin receptors aren't sensitive to insulin anymore, then insulin can't lower your blood sugar.

What happens when your blood sugar stays too high for long periods of time?

Your body can begin to suffer several negative effects. Many people who suffer from diabetes, whether it's type 1 or type 2, endure a variety of health problems. The American Diabetes Association states that two-thirds of people with diabetes will suffer from either a stroke or heart disease. This is because the resulting high blood sugar and insulin levels and elevated inflammatory markers damage the circulatory system. Elevated blood sugar and insulin levels are likely worse for your heart and blood vessels than elevated cholesterol levels.

Other parts of your body will also be affected by high blood sugar. For instance, your kidney function can greatly decrease. If your kidneys can't function properly, waste won't be filtered out of the bloodstream. Because all other body organs and glands will be affected by the build-up of these waste products, this can cause even more health issues. Diabetes damage will begin to accelerate.

Your eyes will also be affected. If your blood sugar stays too high for too long, it can cause the blood vessels in your eyes to deteriorate, which can ultimately lead to blindness.

Another thing to consider is the damage to your nervous system. High blood sugar will result in sugar sticking to and damaging blood cells and proteins, which then causes clogging of small blood vessels. That, in turn, prohibits oxygen and other nutrients from getting to your nerves. When that happens, you can end up with neuropathy, which is what happens when your nerves die. To compound things, many of the medications typically prescribed for diabetics, including Metformin and statins, also contribute to neuropathy due to nutrient deficiencies. Metformin robs your body of essential B vitamins[49, 50, 51] while statins can starve your nerves of the fat they need to stay protected and functioning.[52, 53] Talk about an up-hill battle.

As you can see, serious complications can arise from blood sugar that stays too high for too long. This is why people suffering from diabetes must reduce or eliminate their sugar intake. If you're working to eliminate sugar from your diet and following Dr. Steph's Plate Rule© to do this, please note that you will still be eating ample amounts of complex carbohydrates so your body gets enough energy. You will also be replacing these eliminated sugars with increased amounts of healthy fats, which, it turns out, are a better choice for fueling the body's energy needs.[54]

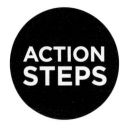

ACTION STEPS

1. **If you're accustomed to eating a high-sugar diet, start by cutting out the obvious sweets—soda, juices, and candy.** Check the label to see how much sugar is in it. Also look at total carbohydrates—complex forms of sugar that get broken down into sugar in the body. 5 grams of sugar on the label is equivalent to 1 level teaspoon of table sugar. You can see in the label below that this product contains almost 9 teaspoons of sugar (3 tablespoons) – quite a bit, right? Notice that the label offers no recommended percent daily value of sugar.

Nutrition Facts
Serving Size 1 container (227g)

Amount Per Serving

Calories 240   Calories from Fat 25

	% Daily Value*
Total Fat 3g	4 %
Saturated Fat 1.5g	9 %
Trans Fat 0g	
Cholesterol 15mg	5 %
Sodium 140mg	6 %
Total Carbohydrate 46g	15 %
Dietary Fiber Less than 1g	3 %
Sugars 44g	
Protein 9g	

Vitamin A	2 %	Vitamin C	4 %
Calcium	35 %	Iron	0 %

*Percent Daily Values are based on a 2,000 calorie diet. Your Daily Values may be higher or lower depending on your calorie needs.

Nutrition Facts
8 servings per container

Serving size   2/3 cup (55g)

Amount per 2/3 cup

Calories   230

% DV*	
12%	**Total Fat** 8g
5%	Saturated Fat 1g
	Trans Fat 0g
0%	**Cholesterol** 0mg
7%	**Sodium** 160mg
12%	**Total Carbs** 37g
14%	Dietary Fiber 4g
	Sugars 1g
	Added Sugars 0g
	Protein 3g
10%	Vitamin D 2mcg
20%	Calcium 260mg
45%	Iron 8mg
5%	Potassium 235mg

Here's a label for fried potato chips. Notice that the "sugar" is 1 gram. At first glance, you could think this is a good snack choice because it's "low in sugar." Don't be deceived. This doesn't make it a safe, sugar-free food. Total "carbs" is 37 grams, while "fiber" is only 4 grams. This means that the rest of the carbs that aren't accounted for as sugar and fiber are starches that will ultimately become sugar in your body. Put the bag down and walk away . . . slowly . . . now turn and run!

2. **Learn to recognize the alternate names for sugar on nutrition labels and eliminate those alternatives from your diet.** Sugars are hidden in the following ingredients you will see in the ingredient list:
   - Corn, corn syrup, corn meal, corn flour, high fructose corn syrup
   - Honey, maple syrup, maple sugar, cane juice, brown sugar, molasses, rice syrup, barley malt
   - Anything ending with 'ose': dextrose, maltose, sucrose, fructose, galactose, lactose
3. **Limit your fruit to one per day at the most, consumed ideally in the morning as a snack** (not with breakfast, which as per Dr. Steph's Plate Rule©, should be protein, fats, and veggies). Don't eat dried fruit while reversing your diabetes; this can be like eating candy. Because the fruit is dehydrated, you may consume much more than you would if it was fresh, so you'll be getting several extra servings of sugar.
4. **Stick to natural, whole-food snacks like fresh veggies and nuts, as this will help you to cut back on sweet treats and keep the cravings away.** If you must indulge in something sweet, make sure that it's something that doesn't contain too much sugar. High amounts of sugar aren't good for anyone, especially those suffering from diabetes.

14

GET RID OF THE PINK, YELLOW, AND BLUE PACKETS—
NO ARTIFICIAL SWEETENERS

Artificial sweeteners should never be used to replace sugar. Our society has been trained to think that just because a food or drink has the word "diet" or "sugar free" on it that it's good for us.

Wrong.

Today, most of the diet products on the market contain artificial sweeteners—aspartame, neotame, acesulfame potassium, saccharin, and sucralose. Reports have linked these substances to insulin spikes, weight gain, cancer, diabetes, headaches, brain dysfunction, and enlarged kidneys and liver. A study published in the *American Journal of Clinical Nutrition* concluded that drinking one 12-ounce diet soda per week increases your likelihood of becoming a diabetic by 33 percent. And it's safe to say that most diet soda drinkers aren't having just one can per week.

There are many other reasons to cut out artificial sweeteners. First of all, studies show that people who consume artificial sweeteners tend to eat more. This is because the additives in these sweeteners often induce cravings. This is also true for diet soda. In fact, many people who drink diet soda are more obese than those who drink regular soda. Artificial sweeteners are sometimes hundreds of times sweeter than real sugar. This causes us to have a higher sensitivity to sweets, which makes us want more of them. The more sweets you eat, the more sweets you will want. It also works the other way around—if you eat fewer sweets, you will eventually lose your taste for them and reduce your sugar cravings.

Research published in 2014 confirms that chemical sweeteners alter the balance of the bacteria in our gut, too. This can cause glucose intolerance and hyperglycemia (elevations in blood sugars).[55]

Our recommendation is to avoid all artificial sweeteners along with the food and drinks that contain them. Your taste buds may need some time to adapt, but the change is well worth it. Use minimal amounts of stevia or monk fruit, also known as luo han fruit extract, if necessary. Stevia and monk fruit are natural, plant-based sweeteners that are an excellent substitute for artificial sweeteners and sugar. Once sugars are in normal range, then you can see how you do with minimal amounts of natural sugars such as organic maple syrup grade A dark, coconut sugar, or organic brown sugars.

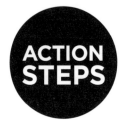

1. **Throw out all artificial sweeteners and foods that contain these diabetes-causing sweeteners.** Stop substituting artificial sweeteners for sugar.

2. **Keep stevia or monk fruit (luo han fruit extract) on hand for when you must use a sweetener.** Remember, these should be used in moderation.

3. **Don't let yourself be fooled by artificial sweeteners and other items that claim to be "sugar free" or "diet."**

Here is a big tip: Cut out the diet sodas. They are loaded with artificial sweeteners and won't help you lose weight. If you love soda and are terrified by the notion of life without it, here are good options for you:

- LaCroix naturally flavored, unsweetened sparkling waters.
- Virgil's Zero soda (root beer, etc). While Virgil's has an entire line of organic regular sugar soda, its Zero line is sweetened entirely with stevia. Kids will like it, too, so these are a great option for getting them off the other brands that are sugar- or chemical-sweetened.
- Seltzer water that you can jazz up:

- Fresh grated ginger, lemon zest, and stevia make seltzer into a natural ginger ale.
- Stevia/luo han-sweetened electrolyte powders such as Ultima can turn your seltzer water into fruity soda without causing sugars to spike. They come in different flavors such as grape, orange, and raspberry.
- Combine Lime juice, lime zest, and stevia into a tasty lime spritzer.

- Kombucha is a fermented tea that's much lower in sugar than soda and carbonated naturally due to the fermentation process. GT's and Kevita, available in several flavors, are generally the lowest in sugars. Most health food stores and now several mainstream grocers offer them.

DRINK HALF YOUR BODY WEIGHT IN OUNCES IN WATER EACH DAY

Water is one of the cornerstones of health. More than half of your body weight is water. In fact, your muscles are made up of about 75 percent water, your brain is about 90 percent water, your bones are 22 percent water, and your blood is about 83 percent water. As you go through your day, you're losing water through perspiration, urination, bowel movements, and other physiological functions.

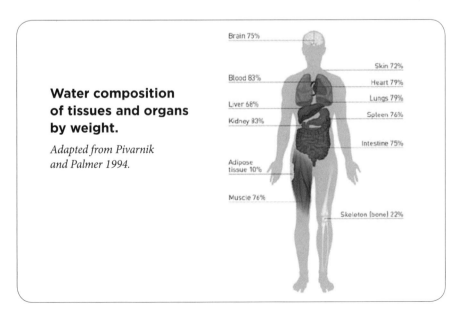

Water composition of tissues and organs by weight.

Adapted from Pivarnik and Palmer 1994.

Brain 75%

Skin 72%

Blood 83%

Heart 79%

Lungs 79%

Liver 68%

Spleen 76%

Kidney 83%

Intestine 75%

Adipose tissue 10%

Muscle 76%

Skeleton (bone) 22%

Water serves many important functions in the human body. Water helps:

- Transport nutrients and oxygen to the cells
- Moisturize the air in your lungs
- Boost your metabolic rate
- Protect organs
- Allow organs to better absorb nutrients
- Regulate the body temperature
- Detoxify the body
- Protect and moisturize joints

A variety of different benefits come along with getting your recommended amount of water each day. One of the biggest is that it helps to promote weight loss. When you drink water, you can lose weight because it allows the body to break down and flush fat through urine. It also helps cut down on your hunger, which means that it's a natural appetite suppressant.

Water can also help reduce headache frequency. Many times, dehydration can lead to headaches and other aches and pains.

Another great benefit of water is how it helps promote better concentration. This allows you to work and think better. It can also help regulate your body temperature, which will help you feel better when you're exercising or performing physical activity. You will also notice changes in your digestion because when you drink enough water, you will have fewer issues with stomach pain, constipation, heartburn, and other digestive problems.

Instead of drinking soda, juice, or diet beverages that are dehydrating and high in sugars and chemicals, drink water. Your goal should be to drink at least half your body weight in ounces every day. For example, if you weigh 150 pounds, drink 75 ounces of water daily. The amount you need can change depending on your current health, physical activity level, and climate.

Some of the common signs of dehydration include dry mouth, headache, fatigue, light-headedness, and thirst. Other symptoms include dry skin, dark urine, and excessive hunger. When you think that you're hungry, you may just be a bit dehydrated. Start the day off by drinking water and aim to drink two-thirds of your goal by early afternoon.

Get your water from a clean, preferably filtered, source. Consider getting a filter system for your house so you can purchase less bottled water. If you want to flavor your water, use slices of lemon or lime, sliced cucumber, or mint leaves. While you may be tempted to use flavor additives, be aware that they can lead to other issues. Most contain artificial sweeteners, which, as we already discussed, can set you back when it comes to your overall health and wellness. You will be surprised by what a slice of citrus or cucumber, or a mint leaf or two can do to your water.

Do you want your body to be a flowing river or a stagnant pond?

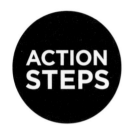

1. **Buy a glass or stainless steel refillable water bottle that you can take with you throughout the day.** If you don't have a water filter system or filter pitcher, buy a water bottle with a built-in filter. ProPur and Clearly Filtered offer good portable water bottles and systems with a filter that removes most chemicals including fluoride. They can be found at www.propurusa.com and www.clearlyfiltered.com. You'll be able to fill your water bottle with tap water but get the benefits of filtered water. Buying bottled water can get expensive when you're drinking as much water as you should each day.

2. **Target roughly half your body weight in ounces in water each day.** If you weigh 200 pounds, shoot for 100 ounces per day. That amount will come down as you lose weight. The easiest way to get this in is to drink 8 to 10 ounces (a doable amount) roughly every hour from wake-up until dinner. This way you'll get it in slowly all day and not have to drink a lot before bedtime, which will keep you running to the bathroom all night. Write down your water intake to ensure that you're hitting your target each day. By cutting out sodas and other beverages and replacing them with water, you will be well on your way to your daily goal.

16

DON'T DRINK THE WATER!

"But wait! You just told me to drink a lot of water all day!"

We aren't really saying don't drink any water. We are saying don't drink the water from certain sources, including your water tap. Here's why:

1. Chloride and Fluoride

Tap water is contaminated with chloride and fluoride and a slew of other toxic chemicals. Fluoride is a known neurotoxin that will decrease your IQ over time. While governments have bought into using fluoride as a method to prevent tooth decay, fluoride exposure beyond the age of 12 has been proven ineffective at preventing tooth decay.

Both chloride and fluoride interfere with endocrine system regulation of hormones. A healthy endocrine system is important for proper function of the brain, thyroid, kidneys, adrenal gland, and reproductive system. All of them help regulate blood sugar in the body. In other words, a healthy endocrine system is essential for an overall healthy body. Chloride and fluoride compete with minerals in the body; that interferes with hormone production and hormone use. This hormone tampering causes reproductive and fertility issues in various populations and contributes to thyroid disease.

Many European countries have acknowledged the dangers of fluoride and banned it from their public water supplies. In the U.S., some state governments are being pressured to give in and add this terrible toxin to the public water system. Fluoride serves no health purpose whatsoever. It only damages brains of and interferes with hormone production.

2. Drugs in the Water

Some reports show that tap water now contains metabolites from oral birth control and other prescription medications. In an interview with WebMD, one expert made it clear that many drug metabolites remain in the municipal water system even after water treatment.[56] The article goes on to say that boiling water won't get rid of these chemicals and that we don't know how they impact human health.

3. Other Toxins in Tap Water

Recently, Flint, Michigan endured a water quality crisis when the local government, in an attempt to save money, switched its main water source from Lake Huron and the Detroit River to the Flint River. As it turned out, Flint River water pollution corroded the city's old lead pipes, which in turn caused lead to leach into the water. Several hundred children are now dealing with the devastating, life-long effects of lead poisoning.

How many other cities with aging infrastructures are flushing our drinking water through old lead pipes?

4. Plastics are Toxic

Some avoid tap water by drinking bottled water. Not only is this costly (in fact, per gallon, bottled water is more expensive than gas for your car), but this, too, has serious health consequences, especially to your endocrine system. That system includes all of the glands that affect blood sugar. (Oh, and as a side note, we're destroying ocean life with the incredible amount of plastic we throw away while supporting "Big Oil"— plastics are made from petroleum and large amounts of fuel are needed to ship water all over the country.)

Don't purchase water in "disposable" plastic bottles and re-think buying large re-usable plastic drums of water. Period.

According to a recent EPA study, most companies refuse to verify the source and purity of the water they bottle. In many cases, bottled water contains bacteria, heavy metals, harmful plastic byproducts, chloride, and fluoride. There is no proven benefit to drinking bottled water over tap water—and tap water is a mess.

In addition, plastic water bottles leach plastic byproducts directly into the water. Bisphenol A (BPA) plastic used in most commercial plastic products is now considered to be an endocrine system disruptor that has been linked with cancer. Heat will intensify the leaching of plastics into the water—remember that the bottles you have been drinking from were quite likely sitting in hot warehouses or endured cross-country trips in hot trucks. Even BPA-free water bottles are likely leaching some type of plastic by-products into the water.

5. It's Not Just Drinking Water

Even if you get a good filter system for your drinking water, you should still be aware that your body takes in chemicals from bath and shower water via the skin and lungs (from steam). And how about when you brush your teeth with unfiltered water from the tap in your bathroom? There's no escape.

What to do, what to do?

The cheap and quick fix is to buy filters you can put on your bath faucet and shower head and to get a good drinking water filter (i.e. from ProPur filters). You'll need to rotate out the filters regularly which can be a pain, but it's doable.

The best thing you can do is to invest in a good water purification or filtration system for your home and for away from home, especially for the water you drink and use to bathe.

Filters can be purchased for the entire water system in your house, or for individual faucets in sinks, baths, and showers. Online stores carry many different brands. Find filters that not only destroy harmful bacteria, but also filter out hazardous chemicals such as chloride and fluoride.

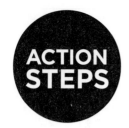

ACTION STEPS

1. **Invest in a reliable filtration system for your home.** You can purchase filtration systems that will not only filter water from your kitchen tap, but also the water in bathrooms. While it may seem like a big investment, it's something you can do to improve your overall health and wellness. If you don't have the money for a complex filtration system, at least get a filter for your kitchen sink while you save for a more comprehensive system.

2. **Get a portable bottle with a filter that you can use anywhere, anytime, to filter out the bad stuff.** Clearly Filtered and ProPur are a good source at www.clearlyfiltered.com and www.propurusa.com.

17

ALKALIZE VS. ACIDIFY

If you have owned a fish tank or know someone who does, you've seen what happens when you neglect to keep the water pH-balanced. When it gets too acidic, algae and fungus grow in the tank. Disease sets in and on the fish—primarily fungal and bacterial infections. Interestingly enough, this is similar to what can happen when humans allow their bodies to become too acidic. They become breeding grounds for chronic diseases and overgrowths of yeast/fungus and bad bacteria.

You can prevent this scenario by eating a diet rich in whole, alkalizing foods and by avoiding processed, high-sugar, acidifying foods. Dr. Steph's Plate Rule© was designed with this principle in mind. When 75 percent of your plate is filled with alkalizing vegetables, most of the meal is alkalizing (raises tissue pH).

Necessary protein-based foods such as dairy, meat, grains, beans, and nuts are acidifying. To counteract that, you need to eat alkalizing fruits and vegetables. Interestingly, raw, un-pasteurized dairy products from grass fed cows are alkalizing.

Other factors that can increase acidity of the body are medications and toxins—and we're exposed to plenty of them.

Why is pH balance so important to the human body?

The human body works on a cellular level. All of the cells that make up the human body must remain at an alkaline pH instead of one that's acidic or they won't be able to function properly. If your body is acidic, a variety of different diseases can begin to develop within the body, including diabetes[57, 58] and cancer.[59] Increased acidity will lead to an overgrowth of bacteria, yeast, viruses, and more.

You want to keep your pH level above a 7.4. When it drops below this, you will become disease-prone. In addition, when it drops below optimum level, your body can begin to store acid in the fat cells and even start to produce more fat cells, which can lead to weight gain.

Another thing to consider is the calcium in your body. As your body becomes more acidic, you will lose calcium. When this happens, you will be at a higher risk of osteoporosis, tooth decay, and tissue deterioration.

So, how can you test your pH levels? You can buy pH testing paper at a health food store or online. Simply place the pH paper in your mouth and wet it with saliva. The paper will begin to change color. Compare the color of the paper with the chart that comes with it to determine your pH level. If it isn't within a healthy range (7.2 to 7.4), you'll want to make changes to get it to a normal range. You can also determine your pH by with similar strips for urine pH testing by dipping a strip in the first urine of the day. Check your pH level regularly to keep your body in balance and avoid many of those negative impacts that acidity can cause.

Another test to determine how acidic you are involves how long you can hold your breath. If you can hold it for 40 seconds, you're in a good pH range. If you can't hold it for at least 20 seconds, you might have high tissue acidity.

Don't confuse tissue acidity and acidifying foods with acidic foods. Acidic foods, such as raw cider vinegar and lemon juice, are very alkalizing to your body, while foods that don't seem acidic, such as meats, beans, grains, and cheese, create acidification in the body.

Generally, most fruits and vegetables (except cranberries) are alkalizing, while most meats, dairy (except unpasteurized dairy from grass-fed animals), nuts (except raw nuts and hazelnuts), grains, and beans are acidifying. Fats are somewhat neutral, but tend to the acidifying side slightly. Dr. Steph's Plate Rule© takes most of the worry out as far as focusing on alkalyzing the body. The emphasis is on getting 75 percent of your meal plate from vegetables with only 3 to 6 ounces of meat, poultry or fish, and snacking on organic fruits, veggies, and raw nuts plus limited amounts of unpasteurized dairy. We encourage eating good fats and oils throughout the day, particularly with vegetables.

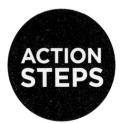

1. Make sure that you're following Dr. Steph's Plate Rule© to ensure you're consuming plenty of alkalizing food by filling your refrigerator with fresh vegetables. When you do this, you will be eating foods that are more alkalizing while reducing your body's acidity. While proteins and other acidifying foods are a necessary part of your diet, they should be eaten in moderation.

2. When shopping for dairy products, make sure you're choosing those that are unpasteurized, raw, and from grass-fed animals.

3. 1 tablespoon of raw cider vinegar after a meal that contains some starchy vegetables will help alkalize the body and lower blood sugars. You can mix it with a couple of ounces of warm water or take it straight.

18

NO TRANS FATS OR HYDROGENATED FATS

For the past few decades, our country has been on a "no fat-low fat" kick. The dumbest thing we ever did was follow this advice. We were told that fat was the enemy—that it clogged our arteries and caused high cholesterol and heart attacks. It turns out that all fats aren't created equal—and not all are the enemy. In fact, our bodies thrive on a high-fat diet when the fats are good fats. While some fats aren't ideal, especially in high amounts, some fats are absolutely vital to our health.

We should avoid man-made fats. These are known as trans fats and commonly found in hydrogenated fats and partially hydrogenated fats and oils. Research shows that these fats increase the risk of heart disease,[60, 61, 62, 63] cancer,[64, 65, 66, 67] gut inflammation (think leaky gut),[68] and disruptions to brain function (depression and bipolar disorder).[69, 70, 71, 72]

These fats are commonly found in processed baked goods including chips, crackers, cookies, margarine, and many other products that have long shelf lives. It's imperative that you read labels carefully, examining them for any signs of these unhealthy fats. Eating them even in small amounts can be hazardous to your health, especially if you eat several foods containing small amounts over the course of the day and over the course of your lifetime—it all adds up. The scary thing is that multi-generational consumption of these fats have been found to create disease processes within the bodies of future generations. What you ate as a child and up to giving birth has implications for your offspring.

To create man-made fats such as trans fats or hydrogenated fats, manufacturers use a process known as hydrogenation to turn naturally unsaturated oils into solid saturated fat by adding hydrogen atoms. This offers benefits for the manufacturers. It extends the shelf life and preserves the flavor. But hydrogenation has terrible effects on the human body. While on the packaging it might look like a healthier option, it's anything but.

Cell membranes are made primarily of fats and various proteins, carbohydrates, and cholesterol. They are a mix of unsaturated and saturated fats, with most of the fat being unsaturated omega 3 and omega 6 fatty acids. The fatty nature of the membrane keeps the cell protected, since fats repel water, while still allowing the cell to remain fluid enough to adapt to its environment and function. Trans fats and other unhealthy fats are brought into cell membranes as though they are healthy saturated fats. The cell is going to work with what's available to it to survive. With a diet high in hydrogenated trans fatty acids, the cell membrane will become less flexible and fluid. That will affect its ability to maintain functioning receptors that allow nutrients to come into the cell (think insulin receptors) and to allow garbage to be eliminated from the cells. If you create problems for insulin receptors, you create insulin resistance and problems with other hormones such as leptin that are also needed to keep a good balance of blood sugar and blood lipids.[73]

Replace these trans fats and hydrogenated fats with healthy, naturally occurring saturated fats. They are found in coconut oil, red palm fruit oil, and grass-fed animal meats and lards (yes, I said lard), as well as in healthy polyunsaturated fats such as fish oil and flax oil, and monounsaturated fats including olive oil and macadamia nut oil. (Learn more about polyunsaturated fats in Strategy 19.)

U.S. law requires that trans fats be listed on label information, but food manufacturers often manage to covertly circumvent this requirement so they can hide the true and somewhat undesirable facts from consumers. By law, each serving of a packaged food product may contain up to one-half a gram of trans fatty acids and be listed as having 0g (zero grams) on the label. Serving sizes are carefully defined in ways that let manufacturers list them in smaller sizes. As a result, the "per serving" amount of trans fats can be listed as 0g. People generally eat more than one recommended serving of a packaged food (cookies, crackers, chips, etc.) as defined on the package. This means that you could be eating food that you think—because of smart labeling—"contains 0g trans fatty acids," but consuming up to two grams of trans fats without even knowing it.

In addition, the types of oils that are generally turned into hydrogenated or trans fats are vegetable oils that already promote heart disease and diabetes on their own.[74] These include omega-6-containing oils, such as corn, safflower, and cottonseed oils. So even though you might be getting lower amounts of trans fats, you're likely consuming oil that is promoting disease anyway.

When reading labels, even if the amount of trans fats per serving states "0g," look further at the list of ingredients for the following: hydrogenated, partially hydrogenated, corn oil, safflower oil, soy oil, sunflower oil, and cotton seed oil. If any of them are listed, put the box down and walk away. Most of the products in the center aisles of the grocery stores contain these unhealthy oils.

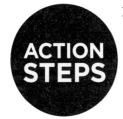

ACTION STEPS

1. **Start reading labels.** Look for the words "partially hydrogenated" or "hydrogenated" in the ingredient list, even if the label states "0 g" of trans fat. Both are clues that the product isn't a healthy choice.

2. **Start by removing items from your pantry that contain trans fat and hydrogenated oils.** Then make sure that you don't buy any more items that include these fats and oils.

3. **As a general rule, when food shopping, avoid the center aisles.** That's where you'll find most of the products containing hydrogenated oils. When you're shopping on the outer aisles, you will have fewer opportunities to pick up foods with trans fats.

4. **Stock up on healthy oils and fats for cooking.** Healthy saturated fats include coconut oil and red palm fruit oil, as well as lard from grass-fed, free-range animals. These are now widely available in most grocers, especially those geared to more natural and organic products, both online and retail. Epic is a company that sells lard, including that from beef and duck.

19

EAT GOOD FATS

Eat good fats and eat lots of them. We know this may go against what you have been told for the past few decades, but hear us out.

The brain is the most important organ in the body. Did you know that the solid matter of the brain is 60 to 70 percent fat?[75] That's right, we're all just a bunch of "fat-heads." All kidding aside, if the most important organ in the body is made mostly from fat, you can see just how important fat is in the diet. Your nerves conduct messages to and from the brain at up to 270 mph[76] because of the specialized fat cells that wrap around and coat them. Without this fat covering the nerves, messages wouldn't be able to travel quickly enough.

In fact, every cell in the body has an outer membrane that keeps the cell's insides protected from the outside environment. 50 percent of the membrane is fat,[77] a mix of both unsaturated and saturated. A balance of both types is critical for cell function and survival, as saturated fats give structure and stiffness to the cell, while unsaturated fats ensure cells aren't so rigid that they can't move and change shape in their environment.

What are the different fats and how much should we eat? We don't want to get so technical that we put you to sleep, but clearing up some definitions will help you understand the oils and how and why to eat them.

You probably know that water is made up of oxygen and hydrogen. In chemistry, the letters "O" and "H" denote these elements. Carbon, "C," is another element. These are the basic building blocks of most living and non-living things, including water, fats, protein, and so on.

Fats are basically chains of carbons—a series of Cs strung together in a row. The number of carbons in the chain, how they are attached to each other, and what other things are attached to them determine what kind of fat you have. Most of what attaches to these carbons (C) are hydrogens (H), as you can see in the picture below:

$$H-\overset{\overset{\displaystyle H}{|}}{\underset{\underset{\displaystyle H}{|}}{C}}-\overset{\overset{\displaystyle H}{|}}{\underset{\underset{\displaystyle H}{|}}{C}}-\overset{\overset{\displaystyle H}{|}}{\underset{\underset{\displaystyle H}{|}}{C}}-\overset{\overset{\displaystyle H}{|}}{\underset{\underset{\displaystyle H}{|}}{C}}-\overset{\overset{\displaystyle H}{|}}{\underset{\underset{\displaystyle H}{|}}{C}}-\overset{\overset{\displaystyle H}{|}}{\underset{\underset{\displaystyle H}{|}}{C}}-\overset{\overset{\displaystyle H}{|}}{\underset{\underset{\displaystyle H}{|}}{C}}-\overset{\overset{\displaystyle H}{|}}{\underset{\underset{\displaystyle H}{|}}{C}}-\overset{\overset{\displaystyle H}{|}}{\underset{\underset{\displaystyle H}{|}}{C}}-H$$

Saturated vs. Unsaturated

The carbon chain, or fatty acid, depicted above is a saturated fat. Saturated refers to the fact that all of the hydrogen atoms that one could stick onto the carbon chain are there–you can't add more. A saturated fat is stiff, solid, and stable by nature. It's common to see this fat as a solid at room temperature. Saturated fats come in short chains and medium chains, and include such fats as butter, lard, coconut oil, and the fatty parts you see on raw meat.

One healthy saturated fat is coconut oil. Organic cold pressed extra virgin coconut oil actually helps reverse heart disease[78] and has been found to help reverse the damage in the brains of those with dementia and Alzheimer's disease.[79] In addition, coconut oil is great for cooking because it's stable at higher temperatures and won't burn as quickly as most vegetable oils.

Now let's discuss unsaturated fats.

If saturated fats are "saturated" because they're completely full of hydrogen, then a fat is "unsaturated" if some hydrogen atoms are missing. Think of it as though there are "empty seats" on the "carbon bus."

$$H-\overset{\overset{\displaystyle H}{|}}{\underset{\underset{\displaystyle H}{|}}{C}}-\overset{\overset{\displaystyle H}{|}}{\underset{\underset{\displaystyle H}{|}}{C}}-\overset{\overset{\displaystyle H}{|}}{\underset{\underset{\displaystyle H}{|}}{C}}-\overset{\overset{\displaystyle H}{|}}{\underset{\underset{\displaystyle H}{|}}{C}}-\overset{\overset{\displaystyle H}{|}}{\underset{\underset{\displaystyle H}{|}}{C}}-\overset{\overset{\displaystyle H}{|}}{C}=\overset{\overset{\displaystyle H}{|}}{C}-\overset{\overset{\displaystyle H}{|}}{\underset{\underset{\displaystyle H}{|}}{C}}-\overset{\displaystyle H}{\underset{\displaystyle H}{C}}-H$$

The example above is an unsaturated fat. You can see hydrogen atoms are missing. Where those spots are empty and waiting for something to attach, the molecule moves around and temporarily "fills" these empty spots by creating a double bond between the two Cs (carbons) that don't have hydrogen attached. The location of the double bond and how many there are in a fat will determine the type of unsaturated fat you have. These fats are unstable and are more fluid and liquid. Think of fats that are liquid at room temperature. These oils include vegetable, nut, and seed oils. Olive, peanut, and flax seed oil are examples. Fish oil is animal oil that's high in unsaturated oils. This makes sense, since fish generally live in cold water. If they were full of saturated fats they would be solid like a stick of butter. This would make it very difficult for them to swim!

Monounsaturated fats have only one double bond, hence the prefix "mono," which means "one." Polyunsaturated fats have more than one double bond since the prefix "poly" means "many." Omega-3, omega-6, and omega-9 fatty acids are all examples of unsaturated fats. Omega-3 and -6 oils are polyunsaturated, while omega-9 is a monounsaturated oil. All three are essential fats, meaning we must eat them every day to maintain healthy and normal function.

Man-made saturated fats are known as trans-fatty acids, or hydrogenated or partially hydrogenated oils. These are to be avoided at all costs. Since they're so harmful to your health, we have dedicated a whole chapter to them.

Omega-3

Omega-3 fatty acids are important oils that must be consumed every day. The best sources are fish and flax oil. Grass-fed beef and wild cold-water fish such as salmon, sardines, and mackerel also contain high amounts of omega-3, as do the eggs from chickens that have been fed flax seeds. Look for egg cartons that specify this–many will even state that there's 200mg of DHA in each egg. DHA is a specific omega-3 that is extremely important for proper brain and nerve function. In fact, 25 to 30 percent of the 70 percent of the solid matter of the brain that's fat is DHA.

The best source of DHA is cold-water fish such as salmon. We ensure that all of our patients supplement their diets with one to four tablespoons of omega-3 each day (see www.MyLivingHealth.com for more information about the products we use and recommend). Another surprising and fun-to-eat source of omega-3, as well as a great source of complete protein and magnesium, is the chia seed. Remember the Chia Pets, those popular animal-shaped clay pots that sprouted? Same plant. Chia seeds are easy to find at your local health food store or natural food market. Add a tablespoon of them to a bottle of water and sip from it throughout the day. They expand, absorbing 11 times their weight in water. You can add them to shakes, salads, and other foods, too.

Omega-3 fats are very important for your overall health. They help prevent and reverse clogged arteries and heart disease because of their natural blood-thinning ability and help the body better regulate blood sugar and prevent diabetes. They're essential for brain and nerve function as well as eye health. Omega-3s reduce inflammation, a major factor in almost every disease, including autoimmune diseases, cardiovascular and heart disease, diabetes, cancer, and many others. Studies show that taking omega-3 supplements during pregnancy helps improve cognitive function and prevent asthma in children while it helps prevent post-partum depression in the mothers, too. This is due to the critical need for DHA during these periods of immense growth and development of the brain and body. Omega-3 fats are such a potent anti-clotting substance that if you're taking a prescribed blood anticoagulant such as Coumadin, you should consult your doctor before consuming therapeutic doses of these oils. You'll want to have your blood monitored and your medication adjusted as needed. A healthy amount of clotting is needed for healthy function.

Omega-6

Omega-6 fatty acids are essential polyunsaturated oils. Some are better for your health than others. Most of us simply get way too much omega-6 in the standard American diet. Although some omega-6 is needed for cell membrane structure and function as well as brain function, too much omega-6 from corn, safflower, sunflower, soy, and cottonseed oil gets converted in the body to fatty substances called prostaglandins. These are highly inflammatory, unleash havoc on your body, and ruin your health—clearly not a good thing.

Because food manufacturers add omega-6 oils to most processed foods and because these oils occur naturally in most grains, we ingest them at a rate of 10 to 20 times the healthy dose. The healthy ratio of omega-3 to omega-6 oils ranges from 1:1 up to 1:4. Disease sets in at 1:10; findings estimate the average fat ratio in the American diet is about 1:24 or more. Not only is a commercially processed cookie or donut unhealthy because of sugar and gluten content, but also it's also unhealthy due to the high amounts of omega-6 fats (some of which are hydrogenated). This is a recipe for disaster.

That being said, there are some healthy, anti-inflammatory omega-6 fats that should be part of every diet. These include evening primrose oil, borage oil, and black currant seed oil.

Omega-9

Many people have switched from cooking with corn oil and margarine to cooking with olive oil. Olive oil, an omega-9 fatty acid, is an important healthy oil and should be consumed daily, but you shouldn't cook with it. Instead, healthy butter and coconut oil are ideal for cooking or sautéing. Macadamia nut oil, which is a monounsaturated oil like olive oil, also handles heat better.

Olive oil is an essential oil that helps prevent heart disease, diabetes, and cancer—just to name a few. It's healthy for you because it acts as an antioxidant, which allows the other healthy oils such as omega-3 to do their job without being damaged. The main reason you don't want to cook with olive oil is that it has a low smoke point. While it might be okay to warm or sauté some food with olive oil at a low heat setting, medium to high temperatures will burn the oil, negating all of the otherwise healthy benefits you would get from using it. When damage to oil occurs, a process called oxidization takes place, which produces free radicals in the body. Free radicals cause damage to DNA and cell membranes. To get its health benefits, drizzle olive oil-based dressings over your food after cooking.

How Much of Each?

Approximately one-third of your daily calories should come from healthy saturated and unsaturated fats. This is easy to do when you follow Dr. Steph's Plate Rule©: Eat mostly vegetables, cook with coconut oil, dress and drizzle with olive oil, dine on healthy wild fish plus free-range and grass-fed meats and poultry, snack on raw nuts, and supplement with fish oil. If you follow the food serving sizes provided on Dr. Steph's food category sheet, you won't have to count calories and obsess unnecessarily. Remember, your body prefers to use fat rather than carbohydrates for fuel, so once you cut out most, if not all grains, you will have addressed many of the causes behind your poor health.

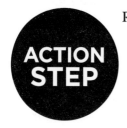

Replace unhealthy fats in your diet with healthy fats. Stock your pantry with coconut and olive oil. Ensure that your daily diet has enough omega-3, omega-6, and omega-9. Also, start taking a fish oil supplement daily.

20

FIND AND WORK WITH A DOCTOR WHO LOOKS FOR THE CAUSES OF SYMPTOMS AND DISEASE

The longer we're in practice and the more patients we see, the clearer it becomes to us how much our society's physical health is ailing. Countless patients come to us with a long list of medications that have been prescribed to treat symptoms (sometimes 15 or more). The average number of prescription drugs that a 65-year-old takes daily is 14.[80] The longest list we've seen had 23. Nobody has told these patients about the underlying causes of their symptoms or how to correct them. They're just given prescriptions as though that's what their bodies need more of.

At best, patients are given vague recommendations that only serve to confuse and frustrate. As a result, they become dependent on medications to treat various symptoms—often for a lifetime. This dependency often leads to a vicious cycle of more and more symptoms that need more and more medication. This eventually leads to a diminished quality of life with advanced disease and sometimes premature death.

Many times, a medication's side effects create another symptom— and the health care provider prescribes yet another medication for that. It's a vicious cycle that's challenging to break once it's begun. We have learned to look for the underlying cause of a patient's symptoms instead of merely treating the symptoms. We work to naturally restore the function that has been disrupted.

For example, let's look at a type 2 diabetic who has uncontrolled high blood sugar and has been given medication to lower it. This person may still have high blood sugars despite that fact that he's taking medication. We often see patients coming to us with sugars in the 200s and HbA1c in the double digits while taking three different medications for blood sugar.

The question then becomes: Why is the blood sugar still high? Before the high blood sugar appeared, other causes for this problem had been materializing as well. These could have been organ dysfunction and toxic overload, cellular dysfunction, stress, hormone imbalances, infections, or many other possibilities. Any of these underlying causes could have contributed to the fact that the patient now has high blood sugar. Since the medications don't address these other issues, the problems may persist even while the patient is taking the medication. Does diabetes medication kill an infection or parasite that may be contributing to the high sugars? Does diabetes medication eliminate a food allergy that may be contributing to high blood sugars? The answer to both is "no."

So, when you're about to choose a doctor to help you achieve your health goals, pay close attention to how he or she addresses your health concerns. It will be apparent quickly whether the doctor is focused on treating symptoms or looking for the root of your problem. Tell your doctor you're interested in finding out the true cause of your diabetes and working to reverse it naturally so you can eventually stop taking medications. Then study the response. If your doctor says "you can't reverse diabetes," or "diet and supplements don't affect anything," think about finding someone else who can be open to and will support your goals.

If you've been diagnosed with pre-diabetes or diabetes, you'll want to ensure that you're seeing a physician or other health practitioner (DC, DO, NP, ND) who will have your best interests in mind. You can generally tell if the doctor shares your approach and is genuinely concerned about your health. Make sure that the doctor doesn't simply write you a prescription to help lower your blood sugar. Instead, you will want to make sure that they help you uncover any underlying issues that may be causing it to be high.

Even when a patient comes in for back pain, we don't just treat it with an adjustment for temporary relief. We investigate further to find the factor or factors causing the pain in the first place. Perhaps one leg is anatomically longer than the other, putting uneven wear and tear on one side of the lower back, or maybe the person's workstation is set up to cause back issues.

When the cause of the problem is treated, the symptoms clear up and the body restores to optimal function. The symptoms aren't simply masked or artificially kept down, only to return immediately once the patient stops taking medications, eating supplements, or going to physical therapy.

If your doctor isn't really proactive when it comes to your overall health, it might be time to look for a new one. Many physicians have extensive experience with diabetic patients. If you're concerned with your doctor's level of expertise with diabetes, you may want to get referred to a specialist. Generally, a physician who specializes in dealing with diabetes will be much better able to help you uncover any underlying causes and will also be able to help you address any concerns you may have about your wellness.

ACTION STEP

Make sure your family physician or practitioner doesn't simply cover up your symptoms with medication. Instead, discuss why the symptoms occur. Instead of allowing the doctor to mask your symptoms, be proactive to ensure you get to the root of the problem. This is ultimately the best way to help you get better. If your doctor isn't willing to spend enough time figuring out the root cause, then it might be time to find another doctor.

21

EXERCISE SMARTLY

Moving and getting your heart rate up are beneficial for your health. But if done the wrong way at the wrong times—or not at all—you can cause blood sugars to elevate. That makes your diabetes worse. There are reasons why we sometimes work to get the patient healthier through diet and supplement therapy before introducing exercise. In many instances when a patient is very sick, we don't let them exercise at all until we have things moving in the right direction with diet and supplements. Depending on how healthy you are, you may want to start working on the other areas discussed first and introducing exercise only after you start feeling better mentally and physically. When exercising for the first time, start out with something that won't add more stress to an already stressed body. Walking is fine and encouraged.

In general, we recommend that whatever exercise you choose to do, you limit it to 30 minutes maximum. A shorter, but more intense, workout is much better than long exercise sessions. This is because intense exercise that lasts longer than 30 to 60 minutes (depending on your health status) can cause secretion of the hormone cortisol, which causes blood sugars to rise. If you have severe insulin resistance and are experiencing high blood sugars before exercise, you may experience exercise-induced blood sugar elevations to even higher amounts. Once your body is healthier and the sugars and insulin resistance are improving, you will be better able to handle longer bouts of exercise. Until then, keep it short and intense.

Walking

If you have never been a regular exerciser, we recommend beginning with walking on a flat surface (or treadmill set to zero incline) for 15 to 20 minutes for at least four days per week. If all you can manage initially is 5 to 10 minutes, then begin with that. Walking outside is even better if it's possible.

Whole Body Vibration

We use vibration plates in our practice to help patients build muscle strength and improve bone density and coordination without high-impact pressure placed on the joints. The beauty of these machines is that no matter how degenerated your joints may be, you can easily exercise and strengthen your muscles without causing more pain and joint damage. The other nice thing is that you only need to use the machine for 15 minutes for three or four days a week to notice significant changes in your body

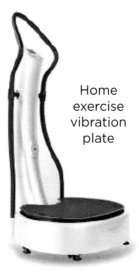

Home exercise vibration plate

and overall health. These changes, which include improved muscle tone, result in new insulin receptors forming. They help your body better regulate blood sugar. You want sugar to go into muscle—otherwise it will get stored as fat and lead to diabetes.

To purchase one for home use, visit www.powerplate.com or www.amazon.com for reasonably priced machines or search online to find a unit that suits your needs and budget. The Axis-Plate E6600 available on Amazon is much more affordable than the commercial machines, but sturdy and designed well enough to create the effect we're looking for. It's one of the best and only pieces of home exercise equipment you need—ideal if you don't have a lot of room for equipment or money for different machines. Between doing strength work on a vibration plate three times a week for 15 minutes and walking four times a week for 30 minutes, you will build muscle, improve coordination and flexibility, and increase bone density—all without increasing your stress hormones and blood sugars.

High Intensity Interval Training (HIIT)

Interval training is another great form of exercise. It can be done outside on a track or in a field, or inside on a machine like the vibration plate or on a stationary bike. This type of training consists of bursts of high-intensity exercise for 30 seconds to 1 minute, followed by longer, low- to zero-intensity exercise or movement for 2 to 3 minutes. This exercise cycle is repeated for 8 to 20 minutes total time, depending on your fitness level. This is a great way to get an excellent workout in a short period of time.

There are many ways your body can benefit from exercise. It isn't just a great way to get your body in shape and help to lower your risk of or reverse your type 2 diabetes. It's also essential to your overall health and wellness. Take a look at the ways that exercise can benefit you.

First of all, you will find that exercising regularly helps get your body into shape and gives you more energy. When you exercise, you will find that you have better sleep patterns, a healthier heart, and even higher self-esteem.

Exercise helps strengthen your heart and improve lung capacity and blood circulation. You also burn calories, which will in turn cause you to lose weight. Since many people these days are obese, that's definitely a huge benefit.

It also helps improve your skin. Since you're increasing your blood circulation, you're able to give your skin a healthier look. This is because it brings the blood flow up to the surface and that helps flush away toxins. You also flush out toxins from the body when sweating. What better way to work up a sweat than to exercise a little bit every day?

Exercise also increases your metabolic rate. It begins to rise as you exercise, but also stays high for hours after you stop. This helps you burn many more calories per day.

When you exercise, you also help build and tone your muscles. Many times, people feel that all they need to do is cut back on the amount of food that they eat in order to have a healthier lifestyle. This is simply not the case. In fact, cutting back on calories and not exercising can cause your body to lose muscle instead of fat. This isn't good, especially for reversing diabetes. When you build larger, stronger muscle fibers, you're increasing your number of insulin receptors. When you increase the number and function of your insulin receptors, you lower sugars since you'll be pulling more glucose, a main source of fuel, into muscles.

Exercise also helps maintain healthy brain tissue and function and has been shown to help prevent Alzheimer's disease and lessen the degenerative effects of other neurodegenerative diseases such as multiple sclerosis and Parkinson's disease.[81]

These are all great physical benefits. Now, take a look at the psychological benefits. First, you will find that exercise helps alleviate stress by taking you away from the pressures of everyday life, even if just for a small amount of time. Exercise can also help to regulate the chemistry in your brain and hormones, as well as energize your brain with increased oxygen flow. That will help you feel better and improve your psychological health.

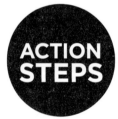

1. **Start with a light exercise program.** If you're not used to exercising, you don't want to overwhelm your body and end up sore and unable to function. Instead, just go for a nice walk each day. You can start by walking half a mile and increasing distance over time.

2. **Get more steps in each day is by parking further away from your job or a store entrance and by taking the stairs instead of the elevator.** Once you get used to walking, you may want to add a few more exercises to your routine.

3. **After you've established a regular schedule for walking and are ready to up the intensity, consider using either a stationary bicycle or home vibration plate so you can increase your workout's intensity.**

4. **Look for a local gym or recreation center with affordable rates** and the equipment you want if you don't have the room or the budget for home exercise equipment.

22

AVOID HIGH FRUCTOSE ANYTHING

When you begin reading food labels, you will often see high fructose corn syrup. Think "corn sugar." Other new forms of high fructose are concentrated fruit juices and agave syrup. Excess sugar in our diet, in any form, leads to weight gain, fatty liver, diabetes, heart disease, cancer, and more. Whether you're trying to lose weight, prevent chronic disease like diabetes, or develop a healthy heart, you want to steer clear of this ingredient.

While fructose has been promoted as an ingredient that doesn't increase insulin levels and blood sugar levels the way glucose does, it still causes considerable harm. The problem with fructose is that when your liver has to process too much of it, it converts the fructose into triglycerides. They are then stored as saturated fats in your liver and other organs. This stored saturated fat is the infamous, disease-causing visceral fat. Fructose may not directly cause insulin spikes and blood sugar spikes, but it leads to deadly diseases like diabetes and heart disease, although through a different mechanism.[82]

According to one group of researchers, "Increasing evidence suggests that the excessive intake of fructose may induce fatty liver, insulin resistance, dyslipidemia, hypertension, and kidney disease. These studies suggest that excessive intake of fructose might have an etiologic role in the epidemic of obesity, diabetes, and cardio-renal disease."[83] Knowing that, it doesn't sound like something you would want to put in your body, does it?

The truth is that hundreds of years ago, fructose wasn't even a part of our diet except in limited amounts from seasonal fruit. It has only been in the last 30-40 years that fructose, especially high fructose, has become a huge part of what we consume.

Fructose resembles glucose, as it has the same chemical formula, but it's metabolized differently. In fact, it has a rapid liver conversion into glucose, glycogen, lactate, and fat.[84]

You will mostly find fructose in bottled sodas and juices. It has become very popular as a sweetener because it's inexpensive to produce. Start looking at all your labels for this added ingredient. If you see it listed on the label, don't eat or drink it.

Not surprisingly, many of the same foods that contain disease-causing vegetable oils and trans fatty acids also happen to contain a lot of sugar, including high fructose corn syrup. You can promote better health by avoiding them.

Many people have opted to use sweeteners such as agave nectar that are marketed as "diabetic friendly." Even we were recommending this syrupy sweetener as a safe sugar alternative at one point because it didn't seem to directly increase blood glucose. However, research eventually revealed that agave syrup is simply a "high fructose" sugar that creates the same negative health effects as the less expensive high fructose corn syrup.

One study showed that consumption of fructose, even more so than glucose, causes fatty liver and impairs insulin signaling, regardless of how much is consumed.[85] A high fructose intake has also been shown to cause increased adipose (fat) tissue throughout the body,[86] cause arthritis and inflammation in people as young as in their 20s,[87] and cause diabetes.[88]

If you have been replacing your regular sweetener with agave nectar or if you've simply stopped drinking soda and switched to organic fruit juice, you will want to cut both out to reverse your diabetes. The only sweeteners we recommend today are small, limited amounts of organic grade A dark maple syrup or raw honey, or small amounts of stevia or luo han fruit extract (monkfruit). The latter two are pure plant-based sweeteners that are sugar-free and extracted from the intensely sweet plants they are named for.

ACTION STEPS

1. Add high fructose corn syrup, common in most types of sodas and candy, to a list of things that you should avoid all together. Carefully review food nutrition labels before making selections. Foods that you're accustomed to eating regularly may have high fructose corn syrup as a main ingredient. Getting in the habit of reading labels is essential to all diabetics and pre-diabetics.

2. If you must have some type of sweetener, **stick to organic maple syrup grade A dark and stevia in limited quantities.**

23

KEEP YOUR POWER ON
WITH ANTIOXIDANTS

All of your cells manufacture a potent antioxidant called glutathione. We need to make glutathione, particularly in the liver, to live.[89] One of the liver's main functions is to detoxify the body, all day, every day. To stay healthy while ensuring the rest of the body remains healthy, the liver needs to protect itself from the oxidative damage caused by the processing of everything we eat and from the elimination of all waste from the day-to-day function of our cells. Between this regular waste and the added burden of waste created from unhealthy foods, medications, and other chemicals and toxins, the overburdened liver does double duty.

Fortunately, the liver produces glutathione, the master antioxidant contained within every cell of the body. It functions not only to neutralize free radicals, but is also needed for:

- DNA synthesis and repair, protein synthesis and transport, and enzyme activation[90]
- Making sure nitric oxide is properly utilized and regulated[91]
- Preventing cancer by regulating appropriate cell apoptosis (programmed cell death to save the body)[92]
- Regulating iron metabolism, which in turn ensures proper oxygen delivery throughout the entire body[93]
- Helping to maintain active levels of vitamin C and E, two other important anti-oxidants[94]
- Helping to maintain liver, brain, gut, and immune system function and health[95, 96, 97]

Many people who are on a path to illness such as diabetes suffer from sick, backlogged, poorly functioning livers. Lack of glutathione allows for increased oxidative damage to organs that are vital to maintaining healthy blood sugar levels, which then lead to higher blood sugars, which in turn lead to further oxidative stress and so on and so forth.

Antioxidants need the help of antioxidant enzymes to protect cell membranes from oxidization and to neutralize free radicals. Antioxidants such as glutathione are more effective when ingested together with antioxidant enzymes. So, if you supplement with glutathione and other anti-oxidants, make sure to supplement with antioxidant enzymes at the same time. This will ensure that you're using your body's antioxidants to their fullest potential.

These nutrients can be derived from good, wholesome food. Nature, in all its wisdom, provides the proportionate amount of each in fresh plant foods such as fruits, vegetables, herbs, and spices.

Other antioxidants that are helpful in reversing diabetes include vitamin C and bioflavinoids, selenium, vitamin A, and leucine. The best place to get these is through food, but sometimes supplements are needed to push the body back into balance.

The following foods contain potent antioxidants.

Berries

The best are blueberries, raspberries, elderberries, blackberries, cranberries, gooseberries, grapes, or any small, fleshy fruit containing many seeds. A word of caution: You must eat only organic berries, as it's almost impossible to scrub, peel, or wash pesticides from each single berry.

Berries freeze well, so you can stock up on organic options when they're in season and freeze them for convenience to use in shakes or salads during off-season months.

Eat fresh, organic berries, not dried berries, which are often preserved with sulfuric chemicals that aren't good for you. Dried fruits usually contain a lot of added sugar, too. This is particularly true for cranberries. When trying to figure out why our diabetic patients' blood sugars have suddenly spiked and remained high, we frequently find the culprit is dried cranberries. Have you ever eaten raw cranberries? They are extremely sour. Once enough sugar has been added for most people even to begin to think about eating them, they have become candy.

Herbs & Spices

Always purchase good quality organic spice and herb products. In general, use a wide range of them either fresh (great chopped into salads) or dried (good for sauces and marinades) to boost the healthy benefits of the foods you're eating. Remember, "food is your best medicine," so adding spices and herbs not only makes your food taste better, it also makes your food better for you.

As you can see, antioxidants are an important part of your daily nutrition. While they are great for those who are diabetic or pre-diabetic, they are also essential for everyone else. It will be easy for you to add them to your daily diet. When you eat foods that are rich in antioxidants, you will find that you also get a lot of other great vitamins and minerals.

Many spices contain high amounts of antioxidants and offer other health benefits. One of our favorites is curcumin, a derivative compound of turmeric. A common spice used in Indian foods, curcumin adds a beautiful, bright, orange or yellow color to sauces. It doesn't have a lot of flavor, so adding it to salad dressings, meat, sauces, etc., adds tremendous health benefits without changing the taste of them. When we add this spice to our morning protein shakes, we don't even taste it. When reversing diabetes and getting already sick bodies well again, we routinely add supplement forms of curcumin in standardized forms to the diet to be sure patients are getting the potency needed.

Did you know that you can get antioxidants in other ways, too? While the foods you eat are the best way to get the maximum absorption of the antioxidants, you can also find antioxidants in many supplements and vitamins in your local supplement store or on our website at livinghealthmarket.com. Most daily multivitamins will contain some amount of antioxidants. Glutathione; alpha lipoic acid; minerals such as selenium and zinc; CoQ10 (ubiquinol); resveratrol; and vitamin C, E (mixed tocopherols), and A (beta carotene) are all good options. These don't need to be taken in large amounts to create a good effect—more isn't always better.

Certain herbal teas also contain antioxidants. Why not replace a morning coffee with a hot cup of organic green tea and enjoy the benefits of the antioxidants, as well?

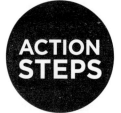

1. **Buy fresh organic berries and snack on them throughout the day.** By replacing one of your snacks each day with food that is rich in antioxidants, you'll ensure that you're getting antioxidants each day.

2. **Buy organic curcumin and add it into your favorite dishes.** Since it doesn't have much flavor, you will get the benefits without altering the taste of your foods.

3. **Consider supplementing your diet with standardized amounts of curcumin and other antioxidants such as ubiquinol, alpha lipoic acid, resveratrol, etc.** Look for only the best quality supplements—those that don't contain fillers, gluten, food coloring, or unhealthy oils such as soy, corn, or safflower. We recommend that you purchase your supplements from a healthcare professional because the products they offer are often the cleanest, purest, most standardized, and best-regulated by the FDA. They may cost more, but with supplements, oftentimes you get what you pay for. We have created a complete line of additive free, bioavailable forms of supplements that you can order at www.livinghealthmarket.com

24

GET THE OLIVE OIL OUT OF THAT PAN!

We promote consuming lots of healthy fats. Many people commonly switch from cooking with butter, margarine, or polyunsaturated vegetable oils to using olive oil. At one time, we made the same switch. On the surface, changing cooking oils makes sense, after all. Why cook with hydrogenated trans fats and omega-6 fats, which are linked to heart disease, diabetes, and cancer?

But there is one significant problem with cooking with olive oil. While it's one of the healthiest oils for eating, it has a very low smoke point. Cooking with olive oil actually burns it, and that removes all health benefits. Use cooking oils with a high smoke point, instead. They can withstand high temperatures, which makes them better for cooking.

Other good cooking oils and fats that are both healthy and have high smoke temperatures are lard and butter from grass-fed and free-range animals, coconut oil, avocado seed oil, and macadamia nut oil. Macadamia nut oil is a monounsaturated, omega-9 oil, much like olive oil, but it has a higher smoke point and won't burn until it exceeds 450 degrees Fahrenheit. It has a nice, nutty flavor, and is wonderful for sautéing and baking. We enjoy kale chips baked with macadamia nut oil. Coconut oil is excellent for cooking as well. It has a nice, fresh coconut flavor and is very good for many functions in the body. We like to use it for stir-frying. Other options for cooking oils include red palm fruit oil, grape seed oil, and sesame oil.

Avoid using other oils, including vegetable, when cooking. They are full of omega 6 fats that won't improve your health. You always want to avoid unhealthy polyunsaturated oils.

So, what do you do with your otherwise healthy olive oil? We recommend making tasty dressings and sauces to pour over your vegetables and meats after serving them. Here's an recipe for a weekly batch of dressing.

Olive Oil Dressing

Mix together:

1 cup of olive oil

A couple of freshly crushed garlic cloves

A dash of sea salt or Himalayan salt

Dried organic herbs, spices, or seasoning of your choice

1/3 c. organic cider or balsamic vinegar, lemon or lime juice (adjust to taste)

You will always have healthier, home-made dressing at the ready, especially during the hectic weekdays, Having this handy will make eating vegetables at every meal much more enjoyable. Steamed broccoli on its own isn't so exciting, but when drizzled with olive oil dressing it becomes tasty. This is also true for many of the other vegetables you may not really enjoy on their own. This strategy helps you stick to Dr. Steph's Plate Rule©, too.

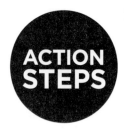

1. **Buy and cook with macadamia nut, coconut, or red palm fruit oil.** Use them just as you would olive oil. Any one of them will help prevent burning your food—and they taste great.

2. **Make an olive oil dressing** to keep on hand to pour over salads or steamed veggies, or to add to morning protein shakes.

25

TAKE TIME TO CHILL

Work hard, but also make time to relax. That doesn't mean sitting in front of the television, though. Studies have found that for some people, watching television can be very stressful, especially when it involves watching negative news stories.[98]

Engage in an activity you find relaxing, whether it's a leisurely bike ride, a walk through the woods, or sitting in the sun reading a book. Take time each day or week to relax. One of the smartest doctors we know, an expert in brain and nerve function, recommends taking one day every week to do nothing; that is, don't do anything you need to do or don't want to do.

If you constantly push yourself too hard for too long, you will eventually crash. We see this often with our patients. Many arrive in our office seeking help to reverse their diabetes or to correct other medical conditions. Not surprisingly, most have demanding professions and lives—they're CEOs of major companies, mothers caring for families, employees with multiple jobs, or business owners. They are clocking enough hours each day to drive their bodies into total exhaustion. By sheer determination and strength of spirit, people literally force their bodies into action each day—they pick themselves up by the scruff of their necks and then drag themselves around for 16 to 18 hours. This constant stress over-works the endocrine system that balances most body functions.

Over time, this hectic, fast-paced lifestyle will contribute to chronic diseases such as heart disease, diabetes, or cancer. Research also shows that stress can impact the onset of type 2 diabetes.[99, 100]

You must set aside one day each week for your brain and body to escape those activities that cause physical, mental, and emotional stress. If that's too challenging, at least set aside blocks of time at regular intervals throughout the year. Shut off your brain and let your body catch up and replenish itself. Doing so will help your body function at peak levels for longer periods of time. You want to be able to continue living well for many years, doing what you do best, with a good quality of life. If you don't take the time to relax and replenish, you'll drive your body into the ground by the time you hit 50 or even before.

Many people have tough spirits with ailing bodies that are crying out for help. Often we see people who have worked nonstop throughout their 20s, 30s, 40s, 50s, and even 60s who have never taken regular time to relax or learned how to implement the lifestyle suggestions discussed in this book. They end up retiring from their careers with failing bodies. The quality of life for many during their retirement years is sad and painful to see. You must think today about the quality of life you want tomorrow, too, and remember to treat your body with the respect it deserves. Your body is the vehicle you use to reach your goals. Take a break, take a breath, and learn to relax.

The most natural time for the body to wind down is from 6 p.m. until bedtime. Our natural circadian rhythms, the 12-hour cycles of ebb and flow of energy in our bodies, dictate that we should be up and running, breaking things down and burning things up, from 6 a.m. to 6 p.m. Then, from 6 p.m. to 6 a.m., our bodies naturally enter the day's rebuild and repair phase. This isn't the time to rev up at a spinning class or put a roof on the house. Activities that cause stress and excitement for the body should only take place during the 6 a.m. to 6 p.m. phase. After you've eaten dinner, begin to wind down and get ready for a good night's sleep.

Start making changes to your schedule and lifestyle today to accommodate time for rest and leisure. Make sure that your busy work gets done during 6 a.m. to 6 p.m. It may be a challenge for the first few weeks, but you will be rewarded. Setting a schedule and actually sticking to it is the best way to ensure that you take time out for yourself. You may have many demands throughout the day, but as long as you take care of them by around 6 pm, you'll have a few hours to devote to relaxation and leisure before you head to bed. You're sure to find that you sleep much better when you take the time to wind down after your busy day. Working right up until bedtime is not only exhausting, it can prevent you from sleeping well, too.

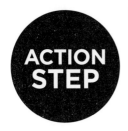 **Find an activity or hobby that will help you relax and carve out a small amount of time for it every day.** Schedule it around the same time every day so you don't forget about it. You might read, craft, or spend time outside. But do something to relax—your body will thank you for it later.

26

GET ADJUSTED

Throughout childhood and up to today, Dr. Steph has been getting her spine regularly adjusted. Since we became chiropractors ourselves, we have been receiving chiropractic adjustments on a regular basis—now at least weekly. "Getting adjusted," along with the application of the principles mentioned in this book, is one of the ways we have been able to maintain such a high level of health and overcome our past medical issues.

Most people know that adjustments are good for improving symptoms like back and neck pain and headaches, but the adjustment is about more than that. The chiropractic adjustment stimulates the brain and nervous system to better regulate and coordinate every function in your body. Adjustments to the spine have been shown to have an impact on organ and visceral function by stimulating nerve reflexes. This, in turn, can ultimately affect how your body regulates blood sugars, inflammation and immune function, brain function, etc.[101, 102]

Spinal adjustments have also been shown to help the brain stimulate and regulate the immune system, thereby normalizing the immune system to function optimally rather than under-reacting or over-reacting, which is the basis for many diseases. The adjustments can help reduce inflammation, but stimulate the immune system to fight when needed in an appropriate way.[103]

At its most basic level, when you have chronic pain that is relieved when you get adjusted, inflammation is reduced. That inflammation's potential for causing increased blood glucose via the stress model is reduced.

We specialize in a technique called chiropractic biophysics (CBP), a comprehensive scientific approach to chiropractic. It combines traditional chiropractic adjustments with postural adjustments, exercise, and traction therapies to mobilize the spine as a whole into its ideal position. It produces results that are more predictable and have much greater positive impact on system and organ function. This approach provides more permanent relief and a higher quality of life for patients. It also results in less likelihood of disc and bone degeneration progression. Proper postural positioning of the spine takes abnormal pressure off of the spinal cord and exiting nerves, which ensure that all organs, tissues, and cells are being stimulated in an optimal way by nerve, blood, and lymph flow. Proper nerve flow to all organs is just as important as blood flow.

Even your pancreas is under nerve control. Many decades ago, medical researcher and surgeon Henry Windsor demonstrated via hundreds of autopsy studies that areas of the spine that were degenerated and impacting nerve health correlated 100 percent of the time with organ disease and degeneration. If the nerves that fed certain organs were being impacted by spinal misalignment and degeneration, then the organs that those specific nerves fed into were also diseased and degenerated.[104]

Many of our type 2 diabetic patients not only have high blood sugar, they also come in suffering from aches and pains. These pains, plus inflammation, contribute to their overall poor health. When we're able to reduce and eliminate these problems, our patients can be more active and less inflamed. This lowers blood sugar levels and increases their overall health.

Many other benefits come along with regular chiropractic visits. The process not only helps you feel better overall, which leads to overall health and wellness, but it also helps correct problems you may have with bones and joints. This could liberate you from medications that simply cover up the symptoms. It can also help restore your nerves, improve immunity, give you more energy, help you sleep better, improve posture and mobility, relieve stress and tension, and address a variety of other symptoms.

Some people worry that a chiropractic adjustment will be expensive. It's actually not expensive at all. Most insurance companies cover the cost, but check with yours first to be certain. If you have to pay out of pocket, you may be surprised to find out just how affordable chiropractic adjustments are.

Others are nervous about visiting a chiropractor because they think it might not be safe. Actually, medical studies have shown that chiropractic adjustments are safe and beneficial. Instead of spending your time worrying that a visit to the chiropractor is going to be risky or that it might hurt, put your fears aside and go ahead and make that appointment. You can ask the doctor about any concerns you have before the session starts. Your practitioner can help put your worries to rest and so you can start feeling better soon.

Visiting a chiropractor is like getting a tune up for your engine. You're keeping everything aligned and moving well. See a chiropractor and get your engine tuned up. You're sure to feel much better afterwards.

ACTION STEP

Make an appointment with a trusted chiropractor (if you don't know one, ask friends to refer you). If you have never been before, be prepared for a pleasant and rewarding experience. It can help you get rid of some of those aches and pains that you deal with regularly. That, in turn, can help you relax and feel better overall. When you feel better, you're more likely to be active. Being more active will have a positive effect on your blood sugar. Make it a habit to visit a chiropractor regularly so you can keep your health in check. To find a CBP chiropractor near you visit idealspine.com.

27

PREVENT DISEASE BEFORE IT BECOMES A PROBLEM

We see it all the time: A patient who is diagnosed with an illness or condition vows to become healthy. At this point, it's an uphill battle, and sometimes that battle can't be fully won. Every day you're choosing to either promote health or promote disease. You're dealing with the consequences of the choices you make. Healthy choices are easy to make; unfortunately, they are also easy not to make. Every choice you make that is proactive and promotes health is like putting money in the bank. Every choice you make that promotes illness or disease is like taking money out of the bank. It may not make a difference either way in the short term, but in the long term, it may be the difference between you living an active, healthy, and high-quality life or living a life burdened with chronic disease.

Generally, pre-diabetes is a warning sign that you will likely develop diabetes if the situation is left as it is. When you're diagnosed with pre-diabetes, you'll want to take every step necessary to reduce your risks of becoming a diabetic.

Ask your doctor for a blood sugar meter (glucometer) and start using it. Many insurance companies won't cover glucometers and the strips because insurers are sick-care, not prevention businesses, and they only cover these items if you're a medically diagnosed diabetic. Making health care decisions solely on the basis of what insurance covers is a sure-fire step to your demise. Inexpensive glucometers can be purchased at most drugstores and online. The meter strips, however, are another thing.

Based on the way that they're priced and the limits insurers put on them, you would think they were highly addictive pain medications. In other words, they aren't cheap. The good news is that there are online diabetes supply stores that sell these items for a third of the cost of most drug stores. It's worth the investment to be able to know your numbers and work to reverse your pre-diabetes before it progresses to the full-blown variety. The worse things are, the harder it is to get healthy.

Check your blood sugar first thing in the morning. Are you in normal range? If not, then start implementing the recommendations in this book for preventing diabetes. As already stated, diabetes is a disease that can have serious consequences when left unchecked. Still, whether you've been diagnosed as pre-diabetic or diabetic, you can reverse the disease by following our plan. Make sure you do everything in your power to help keep yourself healthy. The strategies you've discovered in this book will definitely help you prevent and reverse diabetes.

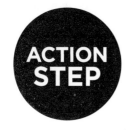

If you're diabetic and implementing the steps of this book, talk to family members about the importance of prevention, since the instructions in this book help prevent it, too. Start checking your blood sugar levels, and your family members', too, and recording them at regular intervals. The only way to know if what you're doing is working is by measuring the results.

If your doctor can't prescribe a glucometer and strips that are covered by insurance, go to an online discount store to purchase them. Search for "discount diabetes supplies." Some include:

- https://www.totaldiabetessupply.com/
- http://glucomart.com/
- https://diabetessupplies4less.com/all-test-strips

28

READ FOOD LABELS

Start reading food labels. This may take a little time and effort at first, but once you do it a few times, it will be easy to spot the ingredients you don't want in your body. Here's a short list of them:

high-fructose corn syrup
partially hydrogenated oils
aspartame
trans fats
sodium nitrite/nitrate
monosodium glutamate (MSG)
food colorings
propyl gallate
butylated hydroxyanisold (BHA)
artificial flavors
olestra
butylated hydrozyttoluene (BHT)
benzoate

Here's advice for reading labels: "If you can't read or pronounce it, then you probably shouldn't be eating it."

Avoiding food additives such as colorings and flavorings is also important. Food coloring has been linked to neurological issues that include ADD/ADHD and autism in children. These products affect the brain and nervous system, important parts of your body that help regulate blood sugar. Even foods listed with good-sounding "natural flavors" are likely to be contaminated with the dubious chemical monosodium glutamate—MSG—which is also a known brain toxin. The term "natural flavors" is a tricky way the food industry avoids listing suspicious or dangerous ingredients with their real names.

Remember, too, that BPA plastic will leech into your foods, so avoid buying things that are stored in plastics or in plastic-lined containers (canned foods).

ACTION STEP

We've said it several times already, but it bears repeating that reading food labels is something that can either make or break your health. When you read labels, you'll learn more about the foods you're putting in your body while you stay away from those that will contribute to poor health. Never buy packaged foot without first reading the label. Instead of focusing on the calorie count and amount of fat, read the ingredients. Buy as many natural and whole foods as you can because they are much better than the processed foods you might be eating now.

SKIN PRODUCTS

We offer several skin cream supplements in our practice. When we introduce creams to patients, they often initially respond with a puzzled look. What many don't realize is that the skin, although it appears to protect the body like a waterproof rain coat, is actually a living tissue that has a tremendous ability to absorb nutrients directly into the body. In fact, some nutrients that would not otherwise survive the chemically intense process of digestion are absorbed very nicely into the skin. From there, they enter straight into the bloodstream and proceed to circulate intact throughout the body.

What this also means is that whatever you apply to your skin in the way of beauty products has the capacity to be absorbed into the body through the skin—good or bad. Most of the chemicals in commercial lotions, creams, soaps, deodorants, and makeup fall under the "bad" category. Earlier we warned about the dangers of gluten in our diet. You also need to be alerted to the dangers of gluten in skin and hair products. If you're gluten intolerant—and that includes a large percentage of the U.S. population—it's important that you avoid gluten in these types of products, too. Wheat protein is a commonly used ingredient in most commercially produced beauty products. Again, read the labels because these products do list ingredients.

We recommend looking for gluten-free products at your local health food store or searching online for them. One of our favorite skin and hair companies, Keys Soap, makes chemical- and gluten-free soaps, shampoos, lotions, and sun blocks.

If you're on a budget, look no further than your kitchen. Olive and coconut oil make excellent skin lotions—coconut oil even makes a great shaving cream. We suggest using olive oil in a spray bottle so you can spritz yourself when you get out of the shower or bath. Coconut oil smells like the beach, so it's always a popular choice. Just remember to separate the skin stash from the cooking stash.

Deodorants are another place you will find toxic chemicals. Even many of the "natural" products contain propylene glycol, aluminum, and other toxins. Baking soda is a simple and inexpensive deodorant option. Make a paste with a tablespoon of baking soda and a small amount of water; apply the paste. Schmidt's also offers natural options, including scented formulas, at www.schmidtsnaturals.com.

Our bodies are exposed to many toxic chemicals. Start to make choices that minimize your exposure to as many of them as possible. Reducing the toxic load on your body will help improve organ function and help you control blood sugar more effectively.

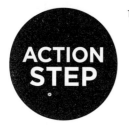

Understand that health and beauty products are absorbed into your body. Get rid of many of the products you're currently using and begin using shampoos, conditioners, lotions, deodorants, and toothpaste that are gluten- and chemical-free. Check the product selections offered by Keys Soap and other natural companies for healthier options.

www.keys-soap.com
www.afterglow.com
www.100percentpure.com
www.schmidtsnaturals.com

CHOLESTEROL ISN'T THE ROOT OF ALL EVIL

The panic on the street regarding elevated cholesterol is reaching annoying levels. The data on which the panic is based is skewed and wrong. Before we get into actual optimum levels of cholesterol, you need to understand and appreciate what cholesterol is, why the body makes it, and how the body uses it. Since so many people are on cholesterol-lowering medications, it's important to understand the misinformation driving the statin industry—and how these drugs can destroy your health.

What is cholesterol? The National Institutes of Health tells us that you need cholesterol, a waxy substance found in all cells, to make hormones and vitamin D and to digest food.[105] Cholesterol produces bile acids to help digest the fats and oils in our foods. It also acts as the main transport system for getting fats safely through water-based blood to every cell in our body, as fat is a major building block of all cells and as a great source of fuel used by them for daily functions.

Like fat, cholesterol isn't water soluble. Cholesterol combines with fats and proteins to form different cholesterol-based compounds that can float freely in water-based blood without creating a fatty "oil spill" within the blood vessels. Visualize a bottle of vinaigrette dressing. The oil and vinegar don't mix. Blood is water-based; fats in food are oil-based. If you were to eat fats and oils and they went directly into your blood stream undigested, you would end up with large pools of oil collecting in your blood stream—and you wouldn't survive. However, 70 percent of your brain is fat and all your cell membranes are composed of different types of fats. So how is the body expected to extract fat from food and make sure it reaches all of the fat-starved tissues while floating in a water-based blood stream without turning you into a big bottle of vinaigrette?

With cholesterol.

The fats you eat combine with cholesterol, a natural emulsifier, and protein. This union enables each fat molecule to be transported through your blood, remain separate from other fats, and avoid pooling. The blood remains healthy and watery while fats move to and from tissues without causing trouble. This is really quite clever. When you understand that one of the functions of cholesterol is simply to get fat to the brain and all cells of the body, you can't help but realize that not only do you need cholesterol, but that without it, you wouldn't exist.

It stands to reason that there's a cholesterol level that would be considered too low for healthy function. The functional range (not lab range) for cholesterol—meaning the amount of cholesterol needed for normal, healthy function of the body, is 150 to 200 mg/dl. Everyone concerns themselves with cholesterol being too high, but many doctors today appear to have lost sight of the fact that cholesterol can get too low. In fact, if your cholesterol is too low, either naturally or due to prescription drugs, then your brain can't function well, your hormone output will be insufficient for healthy bodily function, and your cell membranes will lack the necessary building blocks for health. The integrity of all of your tissues, including your arteries, becomes negatively affected and you actually increase your risk of stroke and disease.

You have probably also been told to stay away from foods that are high in cholesterol, such as egg yolks, butter, and meat. A 2011 study published in the *British Journal of Nutrition* stated, "Dietary cholesterol content doesn't significantly influence plasma cholesterol values, which are regulated by different genetic and nutritional factors that influence cholesterol absorption and synthesis." This means that the cholesterol that you get through your diet has little to do with the cholesterol levels that your doctor is checking through blood work.

According to Uffe Ravnskov, M.D., Ph.D., an independent researcher, too much animal fat and high cholesterol aren't dangerous to your heart and blood vessels. He explains this and supports it with science in his book, *Cholesterol Myths,* saying that the drugs used to lower cholesterol are dangerous and may shorten your life. He also says that dietary fat consumption doesn't impact atherosclerosis or death by heart attack and that there are benefits to high cholesterol. He even notes that people with high cholesterol live the longest.

According to the Mayo Clinic, "It's possible your blood sugar level may increase when you take a statin, which may lead to developing type 2 diabetes."[106] It's significant enough of a finding that the FDA has issued a warning on statin labels regarding blood glucose levels and diabetes. Interestingly, most diabetics are put on statins as part of the "diabetes cocktail" of medications to prevent heart disease. But if statins increase your risk of elevated sugars and actually contribute to diabetes, which is known to damage arteries and increase the risk of heart disease, then might the very medication you were put on to prevent heart disease actually contribute to it in-part?

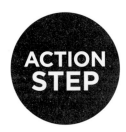

ACTION STEP

Ask your doctor to check your cholesterol levels. Better yet, work with a functional medicine doctor who understands and appreciates the importance of healthy cholesterol levels and will monitor your situation. The goal is to know when you should be taken off them while you're working to reverse your diabetes.

You also want your cholesterol levels checked to determine if they're too low. If you don't take the time to have it tested and discuss the results with your doctor, you won't know which direction you need to go. Repeat this test every three months or so to ensure that you keep your cholesterol within a healthy range. By sticking to the strategies in this book, you should have no trouble keeping your cholesterol in normal range without medication. If you're on medication, then you want to ensure your levels aren't going too low as you implement lifestyle changes.

KEEP TEETH HEALTHY

Several negative health issues can result from having an unhealthy mouth. Aside from looking and smelling bad, an unhealthy mouth can lead to or be a signal of poor overall body health. Bacteria and other parasites can build up in the mouth and eventually make their way into the blood stream—particularly in the case of infected gums. The infection triggers the immune system to attack and cause inflammation. In a diabetic, this can lead to sugar spikes. In a non-diabetic or pre-diabetic, unhealthy teeth and gums can be the straw that breaks the camel's back, eventually leading to full-blown diabetes.[107, 108]

In fact, it's been found that HbA1c and fasting blood glucose will come down in patients with periodontal disease after having non-surgical periodontal therapy.[109]

We had one patient whose sugars came down into the 120s from the 200s, but those levels wouldn't drop any further no matter how well she complied with her program. Finally, after decades of not taking the best care of her teeth, she and her dentist agreed it was time to replace all of them with dentures. Two weeks after her gums had healed, our patient's fasting sugar levels dropped below 100 for the first time.

In fact, many diabetics in our practice have poor gum and mouth health. We have even encountered people who achieved lowered sugars, HbA1c, and cholesterol, only to one day arrive with their sugar logs suddenly showing them up 100+ points—with nothing having changed in their diet or schedule. Upon further investigation, in many of these cases, it turned out to be a tooth abscess or a rotting tooth that required extraction.

When the mouth is inflamed, the immune system is on high alert. When you have any type of inflammation (immune response), especially in the case infection or pain, you will also have elevated sugars. This is primarily because cortisol is released in response to elevated inflammation as a way of regulating the negative effects of inflammation and the stress on the body. Unfortunately, the secondary effects of cortisol release are elevated sugars in the blood and insulin resistance.

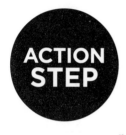

Get regular dental cleanings twice a year so your dentist can identify any potential oral issues you may be facing. Also, make sure that you brush and floss daily. Maintaining healthy teeth and gums is critical to your overall health. If you have any type of cavity or abscess, make sure that it's addressed promptly to avoid further complications.

We strongly encourage you to find a biologic dentist or green dentist in your area who will have a good understanding of how the teeth affect the body and vice versa. You want a dentist who will use only the most natural, bio-identical means of keeping your mouth healthy.

32

BALANCE GUT FLORA

Research shows that your gut/intestinal health affects your overall health. It's estimated that 70 to 80 percent of your immune system is located in your digestive system.[110] Lower fasting blood glucose is noted with probiotic use.[111] Overall, probiotic supplementation to restore good bacteria has a positive effect on blood sugars and type 2 diabetes while improving cholesterol balance.[112]

Roughly three pounds of good bacteria line our intestines, and we apparently have just as many bacteria in our bodies as we do human cells.[113] The friendly flora in our guts protect and defend us from invaders and toxins, help us digest our food, and extract and deliver important vitamins we need to prevent low bone density, hormone imbalances, and brain dysfunction—not to mention a plethora of other chronic diseases. Not only does this flora actively support the immune system by regulating the immune responses in your gut, but they also take up a lot of space in your intestines and physically crowd out "bad" bacteria, yeast, fungus, and parasites, which are also known causes of chronic inflammation and disease.

Anything that can cause this delicate balance of hundreds of species of bacteria to become imbalanced can result in elevated inflammation and blood sugars and ultimately lead to or worsen type 2 diabetes. High amounts of good bacteria keep candida yeast and other fungus cells down. Yeast feeds off sugars and then turns around and contributes to many diseases, including diabetes.

The following conditions can cause destructive imbalances in your gut flora:

- Stress
- Medications, including antibiotics
- Artificial sweeteners and other food additives
- Moldy/old food
- Over-processed and over-cooked foods
- Eating too much sugar and sugar-containing grains foods, etc.
- infections

If you've ever taken antibiotics, you must take a daily high-dose probiotic supplement to help maintain the healthy bacteria population. Antibiotics don't simply kill the bad bacteria; they also kill the good bacteria, leaving your gut cleaned out and susceptible to yeast and fungus overgrowth. You can also end up with too much bad bacteria, such as clostridia. This is why it's common for people to suffer from yeast infections or other illnesses after a round of antibiotics.

We recommend a quality probiotic that doesn't require refrigeration and has a very high count of the "good guys." If your probiotic requires refrigeration, it's likely not able to penetrate and hold onto the lining of the gut very well. You also want to look for a probiotic that has a wide number of different types of bacteria, not simply acidophilus. We also don't recommend that you depend on yogurt for your "good guys." Pasteurized dairy yogurt isn't healthy for you because it generally contains too much sugar, which causes inflammation. In addition, pasteurized dairy doesn't contain enough beneficial bacteria, nor does it contain a wide variety of bacteria (most contain only added acidophilus).

ACTION STEP

Get a daily probiotic supplement at your local health foods store or online at our store www. livinghealthmarket.com. While it's an important part of your daily nutritional intake, it's even more important if you're ever prescribed antibiotics. Probiotics will help to promote the healthy bacteria that live in your stomach and can help fight off many different illnesses and other complications.

STOP SMOKING

It's no secret that smoking is bad for your health and wellness. What many people don't understand is that smoking can not only increase your chances of getting cancer, but it can also increase your risk of many other conditions—including type 2 diabetes.

A little over 10 years ago, researchers studied the effects of smoking on insulin sensitivity. This test involving 40 patients with type 2 diabetes found "insulin resistance was markedly aggravated among those who smoked. Smoking also appears to be associated with larger upper body fat distribution—a marker of insulin resistance, raised plasma glucose concentrations, and overt diabetes."[114]

It was also recently revealed that cigarettes actually contain sugar. According to the Swiss Federal Office of Public Health, the tobacco industry adds sugar to cigarettes to improve flavor and help bind ingredients. The chemical byproducts of the burned sugars have been found to be carcinogenic.[115]

If you're a smoker, you will definitely want to stop. Fortunately, there are many options available to help you successfully quit smoking. The first step involves deciding that you're ready to quit. While there may be many people around you who trying to get you to stop smoking already, you really can't take the next step until you're sure that you're ready. Only you can make the decision to quit.

Next, take time to get ready to quit. Start by setting a date, then stick to it. Pick a time when you won't be dealing with additional life stresses. If you're stressed, you're more likely to start smoking again. Next, find someone who will quit with you. If you have a quitting partner and you hold each other accountable, it can be much easier.

Finally, determine how you will quit. Some people choose to stop cold turkey. While this may work for some, it's not ideal for others. You may want to cut back a bit each day until you have completely quit. Either way, you're sure to find a method that will work for you.

Quitting smoking will benefit not only you, but also those around you. After all, secondhand smoke isn't filtered. Think of them as you improve your own health, too.

ACTION STEP

Create a plan of action to help you quit smoking. While it isn't usually something that happens overnight, if you write down your plan, you're much more likely to stick with it. Also, post small reminders around your home to keep the benefits of quitting fresh in your mind. When you think of lighting up a cigarette, look at your reminders. Consider reading *Allen Carr's Easy Way to Stop Smoking.* Several of our patients have been successful after reading it.

WHAT HAPPENS IF YOU IGNORE PRE-DIABETES?

Here are some of the consequences that may come from ignoring pre-diabetes.

Pre-diabetes is the pre-cursor to full-blown diabetes. Most of the people who end up being diagnosed with type 2 diabetes have experienced pre-diabetes, but some weren't aware of it. When you're pre-diabetic, you have spikes in blood glucose levels, but your body can compensate for the most part, producing enough insulin to keep sugars in a high-normal range. But HbA1c is creeping up between 5.8 to 6.4 percent, an indication that elevated blood sugar is beginning to cause cellular damage.

If you don't follow the necessary steps to get your blood glucose levels down, you will likely end up with a type 2 diabetes diagnosis at some point—a diagnosis that could have been prevented by following the steps in this book. Diabetes brings complications, the most severe of which include heart disease, renal failure, blindness, amputation, and even death.

Most doctors view a pre-diabetes diagnosis as an opportunity to intervene before diabetes comes on full force. According to the American Diabetic Association (ADA), the U.S. has almost 30 million type 2 diabetics, but as of 2012, there are almost 90 million Americans with pre-diabetes.[116] If you're one or the other, you will want to make sure that you're doing everything possible to keep it from becoming a more serious issue.

The unfortunate truth is that diabetes kills. In fact, the ADA says it's the sixth leading cause of death in the U.S. This is alarming news for those affected. Instead of becoming another statistic and letting diabetes end you, end diabetes by taking control of your health. It's in your hands when you're diagnosed with diabetes or pre-diabetes. You have the resources and tools necessary to reverse it and keep it under control so that you will reduce your risk of death due to this disease.

So many people who are diagnosed with diabetes or pre-diabetes don't take the time to become educated about it. This can ultimately cost you your life. Get started by implementing these steps in your daily life in an effort to fight diabetes and pre-diabetes.

WHERE DO I START?

You're probably wondering, "Where do I start?" You may be a little overwhelmed by all the things you want to change and implement.

Take a breath and start as quickly or as slowly as you can, but start!

You can use each chapter in this book as a personal checklist. Implement one thing from the checklist every day, week, or month. Remember, we're talking about lifelong changes. If your poor health is advanced, you might consider implementing these steps more quickly, making changes daily or weekly.

Read through each of these steps so you can learn more about how making these changes will impact your life. When you do this, everything will start to make sense. It may not make much sense at first, but when you take a look at how things work within your body, it will start to come together. After you read through the steps, choose the ones that will be the easiest for you to implement. Start with these steps, but don't let your journey stop there. Making small changes regularly will ultimately help you reconstruct your entire way of living, which can be helpful to your overall health and wellness.

You don't want to consider making all the changes at once, as this will simply be too overwhelming. You will likely find that it's too difficult to make all of these changes, and then you may want to give up. Implementing one at a time makes it much easier for you. Start with a calendar, adding one step each week. This will give you a whole week to master each step. This approach will make it easier when it comes time to add a second step, a third, and so on. After all, a journey of a thousand miles starts with a single step. Sometimes, the hardest step is that first one. This is why the first strategy in this guide is one of the most important. You must get into the right frame of mind to have a successful journey.

Included with this book is an instruction manual for Dr. Steph's Plate Rule©. It's the easiest item to focus on first. Just start creating your meals to follow the Plate Rule©.

Next, look at your schedule. Are you eating a meal or snack every two or three hours, or do you skip meals or snacks and only eat whenever? Map out a set time for each meal and snack. Use the included sample schedule on page 29 for this. For example, if you wake up at 8 a.m., you will schedule breakfast for 8:30 (whether you're hungry or not). From there, you might have a morning snack (according to the rules) at 10:30, then lunch at 12:30. Your afternoon snack might be at 3:00, with dinner at 6:00. This should be the basic outline for your day. Everything else, including work, should be planned around your outline.

You can take control of your health. Keep implementing a new item on this checklist every week, tweaking your schedule to make time for exercise, relaxation, sleep, etc. Slowly begin to stock up on the supplements your body needs. For clinical support, find a functional medical doctor in your area who can run the appropriate tests for you, will design a personal program for you to follow, and will monitor your progress.

Once you commit to small changes, you will start to see your body change, feel your energy increase, and notice improvements in your mood and general outlook on life over time.

Many of our patients experience moments of intense frustration and anger towards the nation's methods and systems of food processing, an unfair and greedy insurance industry that refuses coverage for health issues that truly matter, and a health care system that is more suitably named a "sick care" system. Many of your doctors are just as frustrated as you are. They want you to be healthy, but our current systems don't allow that to happen.

The hard, cold reality is that your health is your responsibility. Relying on care simply because your insurance plan covers it is granting permission to "the system" to take full responsibility for your health—a system that is more interested in dollars than a healthy population (and by healthy we mean functioning at peak performance without medication). Once you realize that your health is your responsibility, you must also accept that you can't blame your poor health on your insurance company, the drug companies, your doctor, or the government, because your health is truly your responsibility.

When you bring your car to a mechanic, you don't simply take his or her word for it that your car needs $800 worth of repairs. You grill your mechanic, ask questions, and investigate what you're told. You should take the same interest in your own health. Learn how your body works and what it needs, then implement the overhaul. If you're going to put premium fuel and oil into your new car, then you must also be willing to put the best quality foods and water into your body. Otherwise, what's the point?

Your health insurance is much like your car insurance—it's there for medical emergencies, not day-to-day maintenance and preventative care. Don't be angry that your health insurance doesn't cover supplements, exercise programs, organic foods, and so on. Your car insurance doesn't cover tire rotation, windshield wiper replacement, oil changes, and new brakes—that's on you. You have the freedom to choose how you do those things. How much will you spend? Where will you go? What products will you use? You absolutely want to have that freedom when it comes to choosing products for your health. When you take full responsibility, you won't neglect to do something that would be good for you just because your insurance company doesn't cover it.

When you take this level of responsibility for your health and life, you can no longer blame the food manufacturers for poisoning you, or the government for approving the process. You have the freedom in this country to choose to be healthy or to be sick. Until you take full responsibility for yourself, you will likely remain sick.

When work, family, friends, or church seem to get in your path and distract you from making the right choices, remember to get back on the right path, avoid the detours, modify your schedules or behaviors, and make accommodations for those things that matter to you. If these suggestions don't work, then consider removing the barriers completely. Make new friends, educate the people around you about what you've learned, or join other groups that have similar goals to your new ones. You will be a better spouse, parent, friend, and neighbor if you're healthier and happier. You will be more productive and able to help and contribute more when you're healthier. So, when the guilt surfaces or you feel an urge to put your needs aside for those of others, stop and remember that the most important, full-time job you have on this planet is to survive and take care of your body first. Only then will you be able to handle the responsibility and joys of helping those around you. You can lead by example. Remember what the flight attendant tells you on the plane—put your oxygen mask on first before helping others.

Take a breath and get ready for an adventure. Consider yourself forgiven for not having known how to become healthy and stay healthy. Simply move forward now into your healthy future with a commitment to a lifetime of learning and implementing things that will help you better understand and become a healthier, happier you.

When things feel overwhelming, step back and take a look at what you have accomplished thus far. Re-read the list of things to implement and get back on track. Take the time that you need to change. The information we have provided will help you simplify and achieve your health goals.

Keep at it! Don't give up! You can do this!

WORDS OF ENCOURAGEMENT

"Well-managed diabetes is the cause of nothing," says William Polonsky, Ph.D., a world-renowned diabetes expert. While it's thought that diabetes is the leading cause of blindness, amputation, and kidney failure, this is simply not the case. It's poorly controlled diabetes that actually leads to these problems later in life. According to Polonsky, if your diabetes is well-controlled, you generally won't have to deal with these problems. Therefore, people who do control or reverse their diabetes can actually have a long and healthy life.[117]

With this in mind, it helps to encourage each and every patient who has been diagnosed with diabetes or pre-diabetes. Many people feel overwhelmed when they have been diagnosed with this condition. They feel as if they have been delivered a death sentence, but that doesn't have to be the case. While diabetes is a disease that does progress if not handled properly, it can be reversed. When you reverse your diabetes, it doesn't have to have a detrimental impact on your overall quality of life.

We have the opportunity to meet with patients each day, experiencing the joy and happiness they feel as they reverse this disease. They have taken responsibility for their health and taken the power away from the pharmaceutical companies. There is no better experience than hearing our patients rejoice that their doctor could take them off of their prescribed medication. These are the results we want you to achieve so you can live a happier, healthier life.

We know many of you have been told you can't reverse this condition. Use this to you advantage, as your motivation to prove them wrong. If you would like to hear from some of our patients, visit www.DiabetesReversalProgram.com. The testimonial page includes videos from several patients we have treated over the years. They can give you the hope and motivation you might need to get started. You can also visit our office website at www.MyLivingHealth.com and enter your name and email address to receive emailed tips and updates. Also, if you enjoyed this book and have found it beneficial, please tell your friends and family. Give them a copy as a gift or lend them a copy. It may be just what they need to take control of their health.

Every year, more and more people are diagnosed with diabetes or pre-diabetes. When you first find out about your condition, it can seem like the end of the world (quite literally). The truth is that it should just be the end of your unhealthy living habits. People who suffer from diabetes and pre-diabetes will need ongoing supervision from a medical doctor, but popping a pill and forgetting about the problem isn't the answer. The good news is that these strategies and techniques may be just what you need in order to regain control of your life instead of letting your diabetes control you.

WHAT ARE DR. CHANEY'S PATIENTS SAYING?

"I have improved my life 100 percent, I love the food I am eating, I am never hungry, and don't have sweet cravings. I will continue this program for a lifetime." ~ Lorraine W.

"My A1C has gone from 9.4 percent to 6.2 percent, and I am feeling better than I have in years." ~ Karen B.

"I am amazed at the improvements in my health. I have energy galore and I feel like dancing!! I know if I stick to my eating plan I won't have to worry about diabetes anymore." ~ Joyce B.

"This program has changed my life. I have a significant amount of additional energy, have lost over 20 pounds and—more importantly— my blood sugar is in a normal range." ~ Matthew P.

"I have lost 33 pounds and feel 15 years younger." ~ Miles C.

"I have lost 23 pounds without dieting, but instead by changing my eating habits and knowing the reasons why." ~ William C.

"I have seen improvement in my weight, my high blood pressure, and my sugar levels." ~ Cora M.

"My HbA1C has gone from 9.4% to 6.2% and I am feeling better than I have in years!" ~ Karen B

"My blood sugar has stabilized and dropped significantly. Tingling in my feet has reduced, I feel overall more energetic, and my BMI is in a healthy range." ~ Jonathan H.

"I've lost 14 pounds, and my sugar levels have come way down. I feel that I have made great improvements." ~ Andy C.

"I have lost nine pounds so far. My blood pressure has normalized, and my doctor has taken me off of my blood pressure medication." ~ Patrice B.

"I have seen great results! My blood sugar has gone down significantly. I am feeling much better than I did just a little more than a week ago." ~ Bernie G.

"My A1C has improved from 9.5% to 5.9% in 2 months. After one month, no more cholesterol, blood pressure, GERD or nasonex medications. My energy, mental acuity and skin are excellent. I've even been able to stop using my dreaded CPAP machine." ~ Jim B.

"In three weeks my glucose has dropped from 278 to below 100. I haven't seen a glucose reading over 137 in 2 weeks. My blood pressure is also under control." ~ David H.

"With the help of this program my sugar has gone from a high of 155 down to 80-100 consistently! I have lost over 40 pounds and my energy level has increased." ~ Barry B.

"My life has dramatically changed because of this program. Previously I was taking Glimiperide and three 500mg Metformin a day to lower my blood sugar levels; now I'm taking no diabetic medications and my sugar levels range from 80-120!" ~ Cheryl L.

"Since I have been in the program my blood sugar numbers have gone from averaging in the 180's to the 90's, I've lost eight pounds and my joints feel more flexible." ~ Larry W.

SAMPLE 7 DAY MEAL PLAN

Day 1

Breakfast	2 egg omelet with turkey bacon, onions, mushrooms
Snack	1 plum or fresh figs
Lunch	1 slice (or half a mini) meatloaf with a small salad
Snack	gluten-free snack bar
Dinner	grilled chicken breast with sautéed swiss chard or beet greens and onions and ½ cup butternut squash soup

Day 2

Breakfast	gluten-free chicken sausage with steamed broccoli and berries/fruit
Snack	sliced apple with almond butter
Lunch	grilled salmon or halibut on a salad
Snack	veggie sticks and ½ cup black bean dip
Dinner	beef taco meat on a salad of lettuce, tomatoes, avocado, with crumbled taro chips on top

Day 3

Breakfast	pea/rice/whey protein shake blended with almond butter and frozen organic berries and veggie/green powder
Snack	pear
Lunch	ground beef with onions, lettuce, tomatoes (left over from night before)
Snack	a couple of tablespoons pumpkin seeds with celery sticks
Dinner	baked cod with sautéed onions, green zucchini, yellow squash and ½ cup baked sweet potato

Day 4

Breakfast	2 scrambled eggs with steamed spinach
Snack	fruit salad or apple
Lunch	gluten-free fish sticks, baby carrots, and broccoli with hummus
Snack	gluten-free granola/snack bar or celery sticks with almond butter
Dinner	halibut filet with rice, sautéed or steamed kale with garlic olive oil dressing

Day 5

Breakfast	gluten-free turkey sausage with steamed asparagus
Snack	10 organic cherries and ¼ cup raw cashews
Lunch	roasted chicken sliced on gluten-free bread (or leaf lettuce if going grain-free) with hummus spread
Snack	taro chips with guacamole
Dinner	t-bone steak (grass-fed), ½ cup beet salad, steamed broccoli with olive oil dressing

Day 6

Breakfast	gluten-free chicken sausage with red/green peppers
Snack	plain coconut yogurt with berries
Lunch	2 boiled eggs chopped over salad
Snack	kale chips and nectarine
Dinner	salmon, steamed Brussels sprouts and beet salad

Day 7

Breakfast	two eggs with sautéed zucchini, mushrooms, and onions
Snack	10 raw walnuts and ½ cup-1 cup of fresh organic blueberries
Lunch	turkey sandwich on gluten-free bread (or leaves of lettuce if going completely grain-free) with avocado and roasted red peppers, lettuce, and a side of sweet potato chips
Snack	veggies and hummus
Dinner	salmon filet, steamed broccoli, and spinach with olive oil dressing

REFERENCES

[1] Allen JE, "Health," ABC News, accessed November 25, 2010, http://www.abcnews.go.com

[2] CDC, Centers for Disease Control and Prevention. National Diabetes Statistics Report: Estimates of Diabetes and Its Burden in the United States, 2014. Atlanta, GA: US Department of Health and Human Services; 2014.

[3] ADA, "Diabetes Statistics," American Diabetes Association, accessed January 26, 2011, http://www.diabetes.org

[4] CMS, "NHE Fact Sheet," Centers for Medicare and Medicaid Services, accessed 2009, http://www.cms.gov

[5] Professional Co-Op Services Newsletter. October, 2005 Vol. 1 No. 4. http://www.professionalco-op.com/pdf/insulin.pdf

[6] Johnson JL, Duick DS, Chui MA, Aldasouqi SA. "Indentifying prediabetes using fasting insulin levels", Endocr Pract. 2010 Jan-Feb.; 16(1):47-52.

[7] http://professional.diabetes.org/content/fast-facts-data-and-statistics-about-diabetes

[8] Bowen, R. Physiologic Effects of Insulin. August 1, 2009. http://arbl.cvmbs.colostate.edu/hbooks/pathphys/endocrine/pancreas/insulin_phys.html

[9] Kim YI. "Diet, lifestyle, and colorectal cancer: is hyperinsulinemia the missing link?", Nutr Rev. 1998 Sep;56(9):275-9.

[10]Pyörälä M, Miettinen H, Halonen P, Laakso M, Pyörälä K. "Insulin resistance syndrome predicts the risk of coronary heart disease and stroke in healthy middle-aged men: the 22-year follow-up results of the Helsinki Policemen Study", Arterioscler Thromb Vasc Biol. 2000 Feb;20(2):538-44.

[11]Goodwin PJ, Ennis M, Pritchard KI, Trudeau ME, Koo J, Madarnas Y, Hartwick W, Hoffman B, Hood N. "Fasting insulin and outcome in early-stage breast cancer: results of a prospective cohort study", J Clin Oncol. 2002 Jan 1;20(1):42-51.

[12]Rosas-Sumano AB, Rodal-Canales FJ, Barrientos Pérez M, Cárdenas-Morales BE, Pérez-Campos Mayoral L, Pérez-Campos E. "Hyperinsulinemia and insulin resistance in children", Rev Med Chil. 2016 Aug;144(8):1020-1028.

[13]Wang F, Han L, Hu D. "Fasting insulin, insulin resistance and risk of hypertension in the general population: A meta-analysis", Clin Chim Acta. 2016 Nov 9;464:57-63.

[14]Harp JB, Yancopoulos GD, Gromada J. "Glucagon orchestrates stress-induced hyperglycaemia", Diabetes Obes Metab. 2016 Jul;18(7):648-53.

[15]Pereira MA et al. "Breakfast Frequency and Quality May Affect Glycemia and Appetite in Adults and Children", The Journal of Nutrition 141, no. 1 (2011): 163-168.

[16]Nishiyama M et al. "The Combined Unhealthy Behaviors of Breakfast Skipping and Smoking Are Associated with the Prevalence of Diabetes Mellitus", The Tohoku Journal of Experimental Medicine 218, no. 4 (2009): 259-64.

[17]Dotson S et al. "Hypoglycemia Increases Serum Interleukin-6 Levels in Healthy Men and Women", Diabetes Care 31, no. 6 (2008): 1222-1223.

[18]Nematollahi LR et al. "Proinflammatory Cytokines in Response to Insulin-induced Hypoglycemic Stress in Healthy Subjects", Metabolism 58, no. 4 (2009): 443-448.

[19]Jankowiak J. "Too Much Sugar May Cause 'Brain Decay'", Neurology 63, no. 4 (2004): 9-10.

[20]Nematollahi LR et al. "Proinflammatory Cytokines in response to insulin-induced hypoglycemic stress in healthy subjects", Metabolism Clinical and Experimental. 443-448.

[21]Padilha HG et al. "A Link Between Sleep Loss, Glucose Metabolism and Adipokines", The Brazillian Journal of Medical and Biological Research 44, no. 10 (2011): 992-9.

[22]Benedict C et al., "Diurnal Rhythm of Circulating Nicotinamide Phosphoribosyltransferase: Impact of Sleep Loss and Relation to Glucose Metabolism," Journal of Clinical Endocrinology and Metabolism 97, no. 2 (2011): 218-222.

[23]Choi JK et al., "Association Between Short Sleep Duration and High Incidence of Metabolic Syndrome in Midlife Women," The Tohoku Journal of Experimental Medicine 225, no. 3 (2011): 187-93.

[24]Darukhanavala A et al. "Changes in Insulin Secretion and Action in Adults with Familial Risk for Type 2 Diabetes Who Curtail Their Sleep", Diabetes Care 34, no. 10 (2011): 2259-2264.

[25]Mandell IB,Buchanan-Smith JG, Campbell CP. "Effects of Forage vs Grain Feeding on Carcass Characteristics, Fatty Acid Composition, and Beef Quality in Limousin-cross Steers When Time on Feed is Controlled", Journal of Animal Science 76, no. 10 (1998): 2619-2630.

[26]McCarty MF. "Toward Practical Prevention of Type 2 Diabetes", Medical Hypotheses 54, no. 5 (2000): 786-93.

[27]Rungapamestry V et al. "Inter-organ Proteomic Analysis Reveals Insights into the Molecular Mechanisms Underlying the Anti-diabetic Effects of cis-9, trans-11 Conjugated Linoleic Acid in ob/ob Mice", Proteomics 12, no. 3 (2011): 461-476.

[28]Love DC et al. "Veterinary Drug Residues in Seafood Inspected by the European Union, United States, Canada, and Japan from 2000 to 2009", Environmental Science & Technology 3 (2011): 7232-7240.

[29]Husak RL, Sebranek JG, Bregendahl K. "A Survey of Commercially Available Broilers Marketed as Organic, Free-range, and Conventional Broilers for Cooked Meat Yields, Meat Composition, and Relative Value", Poultry Science 87, no. 11 (2008): 2367-76.

[30]Erwin C. "Living Well," Livestrong, accessed on 14 June 2011, http://www.livestrong.com

[31]Chiu KC et al. "Hypovitaminosis D is Associated with Insulin Resistance and Beta Cell Dysfunction", The American Journal of Clinical Nutrition 79, no. 5 (2004): 820-825.

[32]Welsh J. "Cellular and Molecular Effects of Vitamin D on Carcinogenesis", Archives of Biochemisty and Biophysics. 523, no. 1 (2011): 107-114.

[33]Parkes-Harrison K, "Public Releases," EurekAlert, accessed February 16, 2010, http://www.eurekalert.org.

[34]Lehmann DJ et al. "The vitamin D Receptor Gene Is Associated with Alzheimer's Disease", Neuroscience Letters. 504, no. 2 (2001): 79-82.

[35]Wergeland S et al. "Dietary Vitamin D3 Supplements Reduce Demyelination in the Cuprizone Model", PLoS One 6, no. 10 (2011): e26262.

[36]Li Y C. "Vitamin D: Roles in Renal and Cardiovascular Protection", Current Opinion in Nephrology and Hypertension 21, no. 1 (2012): 72-79.

[37]Clarke S. GMA OnCall. ABC News, accessed February 22, 2010, http://www.abcnews.go.com

[38]NIH. National Cancer Institute Fact Sheet. National Cancer Institute, accessed June 16, 2010, http://www.cancer.gov

[39]Crinnion WJ. "Organic Foods Contain Higher Levels of Certain Nutrients, Lower Levels of Pesticides, and May Provide Health Benefits for the Consumer", Alternative Medicine Review 15, no. 1 (2010): 4-12.

[40]Alavanja M CR, Ross MK, Bonner MR. "Increased Cancer Burden Among Pesticide Applicators and Others Due to Pesticide Exposure", CA: A Cancer Journal for Clinicians. 63:2; March/April 2013.

[41]Samsel A, Seneff S. "Glyphosate, pathways to modern diseases II: Celiac sprue and gluten intolerance", Interdiscip Toxicol. 2013 Dec; 6(4): 159–184.

[42]Pastore MR, "Six Months of Gluten-free Diet Don't Influence Autoantibody Titers, but Improve Insulin Secretion in Subjects at High Risk to Type 1 Diabetes," Journal of Clinical and Endocrinol Metabolism 88, no. 1 (2003): 162-165.

[43]Serena G, Camhi S, Sturgeon C, Yan S, Fasano A. " The Role of Gluten in Celiac Disease and Type 1 Diabetes", Nutrients. 2015 Sep; 7(9): 7143–7162.,

[44]Johnson RK et al., "Dietary Sugars Intake and Cardiovascular Health: A Scientific Statement from the American Heart Association," Circulation 120, no. 11 (2009): 1011-1020.

[45]Ye J. "Mechanisms of Insulin Resistance in Obesity", Front Med. 2013 Mar; 7(1): 14–24.

[46]Parekh N, Lin Y, Hayes RB, Albu JB, Lu-Yao GL. "Longitudinal associations of blood markers of insulin and glucose concentrations and cancer mortality in the Third National Health and Nutrition Examination Survey", Cancer Causes Control. 2010 Apr; 21(4): 10.

[47]de la Monte SM. "Brain Insulin Resistance and Deficiency as Therapeutic Targets in Alzheimer's Disease", Curr Alzheimer Res. 2012 Jan; 9(1): 35–66.

[48]Marín-Juez R, Jong-Raadsen S, Yang S, Spaink HP. "Hyperinsulinemia induces insulin resistance and immune suppression via Ptpn6/Shp1 in zebrafish", J Endocrinol. 2014 Aug;222(2):22941.

[49]Moore EM, Mander AG, Ames D, Kotowicz MA, Carne RP, Brodaty H, et al. "Increased Risk of Cognitive Impairment in Patients With Diabetes Is Associated With Metformin", Diabetes Care 2013;36:2981–2987 -

[50]Chen Y, Zhou K, Wang R, Liu Y, Kwak YD, Ma T, Thompson RC, Zhao Y, Smith L, Gasparini L, Luo Z, Xu H, Liao FF. "Antidiabetic drug metformin (GlucophageR) increases biogenesis of Alzheimer's amyloid peptides via up-regulating BACE1 transcription", Proc Natl Acad Sci U S A. 2009 Mar 10; 106(10):3907-12.

[51]Wile DJ, Toth C. "Metformin use increase the risk of diabetic neuropathy", Scientific sessions, American Academy of Neurology. April 29, 2009.

[52]Murinson, BB, Haughey NJ, Maragakis NJ. "Selected statins produce rapid spinal motor neuron loss in vitro", BMC Musculoskelet Disord. 2012; 13: 100.

[53]Golomb BA, Evans MA. "Statin adverse effects: A review of the literature and evidence for a Mitochondrial Mechanism", Am J Cardiovasc Drugs. 2008; 8(6): 373–418.

[54]Paoli A, Rubini A, Volek JS, Grimaldi KA. "Beyond weight loss: a review of the therapeutic uses of very-low-carbohydrate (ketogenic) diets", Eur J Clin Nutr. 2013 Aug; 67(8): 789–796.

[55]Suez J, Korem T, Zeevi D, Zilberman-Schapira G, Thaiss CA, Maza O, Israeli D, Zmora N, Gilad S, Weinberger A, Kuperman Y, Harmelin A,Kolod-kin-Gal I, Shapiro H, Halpern Z, Segal E, Elinav E. "Artificial sweeteners induce glucose intolerance by altering gut microbiota", Nature. 2014 Oct 9;514(7521):181-6.

[56]http://www.webmd.com/a-to-z-guides/features/drugs-in-our-drinking-water?page=3

[57]Herter CA. "The acid intoxication of diabetes in its relation to prognosis", J Exp Med. 1901 Oct 1;5(6):617-33.

[58]Shariati-Bafghi SE, Nosrat-Mirshekarlou E, Karamati M, Rashidkhani B, "Higher dietary acidity is associated with lower bone mineral density in postmenopausal Iranian women, independent of dietary calcium intake", Int J Vitam Nutr Res. 2014;84(3-4):206-17.

[59]Sartori HE. "Nutrients and cancer: an introduction to cesium therapy", Pharmacol Biochem Behav. 1984;21 Suppl 1:7-10.

[60]Karbowska J, Kochan Z. "Trans-fatty acids-effects on coronary artery disease", Pol Merkur Lekarski. 2011 Jul;31(181):56-9.

[61]Benatar JR, Gladding P, White HD, Zeng I, Stewart RA. "Trans-fatty acids in New Zealand patients with coronary artery disease", Eur J Cardiovasc Prev Rehabil. 2011 Aug;18(4):615-20.

[62]Remig V, Franklin B, Margolis S, Kostas G, Nece T, Street J. "Nutritional related cardiovascular risk factors in patients with coronary artery disease in Iran: a case-control study", CNutr J. 2010 Dec 26;9:70.

[63]Amani R, Noorizadeh M, Rahmanian S, Afzali N, Haghighizadeh MH. "Trans fats in America: a review of their use, consumption, health implications and regulation", J Am Diet Assoc. 2010 Apr;110(4):585-92.

[64]Barcelos RC, Vey LT, Segat HJ, Roversi K, Roversi K, Dias VT, Trevizol F, Kuhn FT, Dolci GS, Pase CS, Piccolo J, Veit JC, Emanuelli T, Luz SC, Bürger ME. "Cross-generational trans fat intake exacerbates UV radiation-induced damage in rat skin", Food Chem Toxicol. 2014 Jul;69:38-45.

[65]Wang J, John EM, Horn-Ross PL, Ingles SA. "Dietary fat, cooking fat, and breast cancer risk in a multiethnic population", Nutr Cancer. 2008;60(4):492-504.

[66]Qiu W, Lu H, Qi Y, Wang X. "Dietary fat intake and ovarian cancer risk: a meta-analysis of epidemiological studies", Oncotarget. 2016 Apr 22.

[67]Charbonneau B1, O'Connor HM, Wang AH, Liebow M, Thompson CA, Fredericksen ZS, Macon WR, Slager SL, Call TG, Habermann TM, Cerhan JR. "Trans fatty acid intake is associated with increased risk and n3 fatty acid intake with reduced risk of non-hodgkin lymphoma", J Nutr. 2013 May;143(5):672-81.

[68]Okada Y, Tsuzuki Y, Ueda T, Hozumi H, Sato S, Hokari R, Kurihara C, Watanabe C, Tomita K, Komoto S, Kawaguchi A, Nagao S, Miura S. "Trans fatty acids in diets as a precipitating factor of gut inlfammation?", J Gastroenterol Hepatol. 2013 Dec;28 Suppl 4:29-32.

[69]Ginter E, Simko V. "New data on harmful effects of trans-fatty acids." Bratisl Lek Listy. 2016;117(5):251-3.

[70]Dias VT, Trevizol F, Barcelos RC, Kunh FT, Roversi K, Roversi K, Schuster AJ, Pase CS, Golombieski R, Emanuelli T, Bürger ME. " Lifelong consumption of trans fatty acids promotes striatal impairments on $Na(+)/K(+)$ ATPase and BDNF mRNA expression in an animal model of mania", Brain Res Bull. 2015 Sep;118:78-81.

[71]Misan V, Estato V, de Velasco PC, Spreafico FB, Magri T, Dos Santos RM, Fragoso T, Souza AS, Boldarine VT, Bonomo IT, Sardinha FL, Oyama LM, Tibiriçá E, Tavares do Carmo Md. "Interesterified fat or palm oil as substitutes for partially hydrogenated fat during the perinatal period produces period changes in the brain fatty acids profile and increases leukocyte-endothelial interactions in the cerebral microcirculation from the male offspring in adult life", Brain Res. 2015 Aug 7;1616:123-33.

[72]Trevizol F, Roversi K, Dias VT, Roversi K, Barcelos RC, Kuhn FT, Pase CS, Golombieski R, Veit JC, Piccolo J, Pochmann D, Porciúncula LO,Emanuelli T, Rocha JB, Bürger ME. "Cross-generational trans fat intake facilitates mania-like behavior: oxidative and molecular markers in brain cortex," Neuroscience. 2015 Feb 12;286:353-63.

[73]Heshka JT, Jones PJ. "A role for dietary fat in leptin receptor, OB-Rb, function", Life Sci. 2001 Jul 20;69(9):987-1003.

[74]G. Cascio, G. Schiera, I. Di Liegro. "Dietary Fatty Acids in Metabolic Syndrome, Diabetes, and Cardiovascular Diseases," Current Diabetes Reviews 8, no. 1 (2012): 2-17.

[75]Chang CY, Ke DS, Chen JY. "Essential fatty acids and human brain", Acta Neurol Taiwan. 2009 Dec;18(4):231-41.

[76]http://scienceline.ucsb.edu/getkey.php?key=1950

[77]http://scienceline.ucsb.edu/getkey.php?key=1950

[78]Babu AS, Veluswamy SK, Arena R, Guazzi M, Lavie CJ. "Virgin coconut oil and its potential cardioprotective effects", Postgrad Med. 2014 Nov;126(7):76-83.

[79]Fernando WM, Martins IJ, Goozee KG, Brennan CS, Jayasena V, Martins RN. "The role of dietary coconut oil for the prevention and treatment of Alzheimer's disease: potential mechanisms of action", Br J Nutr. 2015 Jul 14;114(1):1-14.

[80]https://www.ascp.com/articles/about-ascp/ascp-fact-sheet

[81]Tay L, Lim WS, Chan M, Ali N, Chong MS. "A combined cognitive stimulation and physical exercise programme (MINDVital) in early dementia: differential effects on single- and dual-taks gaitperformance", Gerontology. 2016 Feb 26.

[82]V. S. Malik, and F. B. Hu, "Sweeteners and Risk of Obesity and Type 2 Diabetes: The Role of Sugar-sweetened Beverages," Current Diabetes Reports 12, no. 2 (2012): 195-203.

[83]M. Kretowicz at al., "The Impact of Fructose on Renal Function and Blood Pressure," International Journal of Nephrology 315879 (2011).

[84]Tappy L, "Metabolic Effects of Fructose and the Worldwide Increase in Obesity," Physiological Review 90, no. 1 (2010): 23-46.

[85]Baena M, Sangüesa G, Dávalos A, Latasa MJ, Sala-Vila A, Sánchez RM, Roglans N, Laguna JC, Alegret M. "Fructose, but not glucose, impairs insulin signaling in the three major insulin-sensitive tissues", Sci Rep. 2016 May 19;6:26149.

[86]Zubiría MG, Alzamendi A, Moreno G, Rey MA, Spinedi E, Giovambattista A. "Long-term fructose intake increases adipogenic potential: Evidence of direct effects of fructose on adipocyte precursor cells", Nutrients. 2016 Apr 2;8(4).

[87]DeChristopher LR, Uribarri J, Tucker KL. "Intake of high-fructose corn syrup sweeted soft drinks, fruit drinks and apple juice is associated with prevalent arthritis in US adults, aged 20-30 years", Nutr Diabetes. 2016 Mar 7;6.

[88]Lozano I, Van der Werf R, Bietiger W, Seyfritz E, Peronet C, Pinget M, Jeandidier N, Maillard E, Marchioni E, Sigrist S, Dal S. " High-fructose and high-fat diet-induced disorders in rats: impact on diabetes risk, hepatic and vascular complications", Nutr Metab (Lond). 2016 Feb 25;13:15.

[89]Chen Y, Yang Y, Miller ML, Shen D; Shertzed HG, Stringer KF, Wang, B, Schneider SN, Nebert DW, Dalton TP. "Hepatocyte-specific Gclc deletion leads to rapid onset of steatosis with mitochondrial injury and liver failure." Hepatology. 2007; 45 (5): 1118–28.

[90]Dringen R. "Metabolism and functions of glutathione in brain". Progress in Neurobiology. 2000 Dec 01;62(6): 649–671.

[91]Clementi E, Smith GC, Howden M, Dietrich S, Bugg S, O'Connell MJ, Goldsbrough PB, Cobbett CS. (1999). "Phytochelatin synthase genes from Arabidopsis and the yeastSchizosaccharomyces pombe". The Plant cell. 199911 (6): 1153–64.

[92]Hall AG. "Review: The role of glutathione in the regulation of apoptosis". European Journal of Clinical Investigation. 1999 March 1; 29 (3): 238–245. ISSN 0014-2972.

[93]Kumar C, et al. "Glutathione revisited: a vital function in iron metabolism and ancillary role in thiol-redox control." The EMBO Journal . 2011;30: 2044–2056.

[94]Hughes RE . "Reduction of dehydroascorbic acid by animal tissues." Nature 1964;203 (4949): 1068–9.

[95]Janáky R, Ogita K, Pasqualotto B A, Bains JS, Oja SS, Yoneda Y, Shaw CA. (1999-09-01)."Glutathione and signal transduction in the mammalian CNS". Journal of Neurochemistry. 1999 Sept 01;73 (3): 889–902.

[96]Sies, Helmut (1999-11-01). "Glutathione and its role in cellular functions". Free Radical Biology and Medicine 1999 Nov 01;27 (9–10): 916–921.

[97]Steullet P, Neijt HC, Cuénod M, Do KQ. "Synaptic plasticity impairment and hypofunction of NMDA receptors induced by glutathione deficit: Relevance to schizophrenia." Neuroscience 2006;137 (3): 807–819.

[98]https://www.psychologytoday.com/blog/why-we-worry/201206/the-psychological-effects-tv-news

[99]Wiernik E, Nabi H, Thomas F, Pannier B, Hanon O, Simon T, Simon JM, Danchin N, Limosin F, Czernichow S, Lemogne C. Association between current percieved stress and incident diabetes is dependent on occupational status: Evidence from the IPC cohort study", Diabetes Metab. 2016 Mar 4.

[100]Walker RJ, Strom Williams J, Egege LE. "Influence of race, ethnicity and social determinants of health on diabetes outcomes", Am J Med Sci. 2016 Apr;351(4):366-73.,

[101]Sato A. "The reflex effects of spinal somatic nerve stimulation on visceral functionJ Manipulative Physiol Ther. 1992 Jan;15(1):57-61. The reflex effects of spinal somatic nerve stimulation on visceral function.

[102]Pikalov AA, Kharin VV. "Use of spinal manipulative therapy in the treatment of duodenal ulcer: a pilot study", J Manipulative Physiol Ther. 1994 Jun;17(5):310-3.

[103]Teodorczyk-Injeyan JA, Injeyan HS, Ruegg R. "Spinal Manipulative Therapy Reduces Inflammatory Cytokines but Not Substance P Production in Normal Subjects ", Journal of Manipulative and Physiological Therapeutics. 2006 Jan; 29(1):14-21

[104]Winsor H. "Sympathetic segmental disturbances. The evidence of the association in dissected cadavers of visceral disease with vertebrae deformities of the same sympathetic segment". New York Med Times Nov 1921;XLIX(ii):267-271.

[105]http://www.nhlbi.nih.gov/health/health-topics/topics/hbc.

[106]http://www.mayoclinic.org/diseases-conditions/high-blood-cholesterol/in-depth/statin-side-effects/art-20046013

[107]Xu R, Zeng G, Wang S, Tao H, Ren L, Zhang Z, Zhang Q, Zhao J, Gao J, Li D. "Periodontitis promotes the diabetic development of obese rat via miR-147 induced classic macrophage activation", Biomed Pharmacother. 2016 Aug 9;83:892-897.

[108]Scannapieco FA, Cantos A. "Oral inflammation and infection, and chronic medical diseases: implications for the elderly", Periodontol 2000. 2016 Oct;72(1):153-75.

[109]Teshome A, Yitayeh A. "The effect of periodontal therapy on glycemic control and fasting plasma glucose level in type 2 diabetic patients: systematic review and meta-analyis", BMC Oral Health. 2016 Jul 30;17(1):31.

[110]Vighi G, Marcucci F, L, Di Cara G, Frati F. "Allergy and the gastrointestinal system", Clin Exp Immunol. 2008 Sep; 153(Suppl 1): 3–6.

[111]Samah S, Ramasamy K, Lim SM, Neoh CF. "Probiotics for the management of type 2 diabetes mellitus: A systematic review and meta-analysis", Diabetes Res Clin Pract. 2016 Aug;118:172-82.

[112]Li C, Li X, Han H, Cui H, Peng M, Wang G, Wang Z. "Effect of probiotics on metabolic profiles in type 2 diabetes mellitus: a meta-analysis of randomized controlled trials", Medicine (Baltimore). 2016 Jun;95(26)

[113]http://www.nature.com/news/scientists-bust-myth-that-our-bodies-have-more-bacteria-than-human-cells-1.19136

[114]D. Haire-Joshu, R. E. Glasgow, and T. L. Tibbs, "Smoking and Diabetes," Diabetes Care 22, no. 11 (1999): 1887-1898.

[115]http://www.bag.admin.ch/themen/drogen/00041/00618/13196/13197/index.html?lang=en

[116]http://www.diabetes.org/diabetes-basics/statistics/?referrer=https://www.google.com/

[117]Boschert S. "Use Behaviorial Strategies to Help Manage Diabetes," Clinical Psychiatry News 65 (May 2008).

APPENDIX A: FOOD LIST

Remember to follow Dr. Steph's Plate Rule for choosing where to put these foods. The top 3 categories (meats and veggies) generally go on your Meal Plates (along with the oils), while the Beans, Fruits and Nuts or combos of these foods generally get eaten for snacks. There may be several foods that have not been listed, simply drop them into the appropriate category and work into plate.

CONCENTRATED PROTEIN

Average size 3-6 oz.
1 serving = 150 calories
Cooked or as indicated (grilled, baked, roasted, poached, sautéed, stir-fried).
All fish should be wild, poultry free- range and red meat grass-fed.

Beef, Lamb, Venison, Buffalo/Bison, Veal, Goat, Salmon, Cod, Halibut, Rainbow Trout, Red Snapper, Sardines, Swordfish, Whitefish, White and Yellow Perch, Yellowtail, Albacore (Tuna), Anchovy, Flounder, Grouper, Haddock, Mahi- mahi, Pickerel, Sea Bass, Sea Trout, Scallops, crab, lobster, shrimp, etc. Chicken, Turkey, Cornish Hen, Duck, Quail Eggs (2-4 per week)

BEANS AND LEGUMES

Ideally from dried and soaked 24-48 hrs.
Average serving size = 1/2 cup
1 serving = 110 calories
Eat for snacks
(dips, cooked, raw, humus).

Adzuki beans, pinto beans, black-eyed peas, Black beans, broad beans, fava beans, garbanzo beans, green beans, lima beans, northern beans, red beans, string beans, white beans, green peas, pea pods

GRAINS/BREADS

Average Serving Size = 1/2 cup cooked
Approx 75-100 calories
Servings—0-1 per day
Best as or with snack, or instead of starch veggie at a meal.

Rice, millet, quinoa (1/4-1/2 cup cooked)
Rice cake or wrap (gluten-free) (1)
Rice crackers (5-10)
Gluten-Free flours
**if you eat grains, and sugars go up, they are out.

BEVERAGES

Water, Seltzer, Herbal (peppermint, chamomile, etc.) - unlimited
Green tea (unless spikes sugar/BP)
Kombucha

STARCH VEGGIES

Average Serving Size = 1/2 cup
Approx 45 calories
Servings—0-2 per day

Sweet Potato, Pumpkin Turnips, Avocado, Beets, Carrots, Yams, All other squashes, Taro root
**kept white potato off the list because this is one of the worst culprits for spiking blood sugar.

OILS

Average Serving Size = 1 Teaspoon
Approx 40 calories
Servings—4-7 per day
All oils should be organic, cold-pressed, extra virgin.

Olive Oil (don't cook with)
Flax Oil (don't cook with)
Fish Oil (don't cook with)
Coconut Oil (ok to cook with)
Sesame Oil (ok for cooking)
Macadamia Nut Oil (ok to cook)
Grape seed Oil (ok to cook)

DAIRY

Average Serving Size:
2oz or 1/2 cup shredded
Approx 80-150 calories
Servings—0-1 per day
None for African Decent

Choose unpasteurized from Grass-Fed cows or goats i.e. cheese, yogurts, butter, cream, milk

CONDIMNETS/SPICE

Cayenne, curry, dulse, kelp, turmeric, carob, allspice, anise, arrowroot, basil, bay leaf, cardamom, chives, clove, coriander, cream of tartar, cumin, dill, garlic, plain gelatin, horseradish, marjoram, mint, miso, dry mustard, paprika, red pepper flakes, peppercorn, peppermint, rosemary, saffron, sage, sea salt, savory, spearmint, tamari, tapioca, tarragon, thyme, wintergreen. Sweetener: stevia, Grade A Organic Maple syrup—limited.

STICKS & LEAVES VEGGIES

Average Serving Size = 1/2 cup
10-25 calories, Servings—Unlimited

Artichoke, Arugula, Asparagus, Broccoli, Brussels' Sprouts, Cabbage, Celery, Cucumber, Fiddlehead Ferns, Ginger, Greens (collards, kale, chards, beet or turnip greens, spinach, dandelion, parsley), Fennel, Lettuces, Mushrooms, Okra, Onions, Peppers, Radicchio, Radishes, All Sprouts, Tomato, Watercress, Zucchini, Green Olives

**Beans and corn are not veggies. Corn is a grain. Beans are in Legume section. Ok for snacks, keep off meals

FRUITS

1 Serving Approx 80 calories
Servings—1 per day
Fresh or Frozen Organic

**No dried fruit—will spike sugars
**No Fruit Juice—will spike sugars
Apple, 1 medium
Apricot, 3 med
Berries: 1 cup blueberries, raspberries or blackberries
Banana (1/2 large or 1 small)
Cherries, 10
Figs (2)
Grapefruit, 1 whole
Grapes, 15
Mango, 1/2 med
Nectarine (1)
Orange (1 large, 2 small)
Peaches, 2 small
Pear, 1 med
Pineapple (1/2 cup)
Plum (2 small)
Watermelon (2 cups)
Lemons/Limes

NUTS AND SEEDS
Approx 100 calories *Servings—1-2 per day*
Walnuts, Cashew 7-8 Pumpkin seeds, 2 Tbs Almond, Pecan, Hazelnut: 10-12 Macadamia, 7-8 Sesame, Pine nut, 2 Tbsp Nut butters (almond, cashew, etc): 1 Tbsp